CAMBRIDGE PUBLIC HEALTH SERIES

UNDER THE EDITORSHIP OF

G. S. GRAHAM-SMITH, M.D., F.R.S., *Reader in Preventive Medicine, Cambridge and Secretary to the Sub-Syndicate for Tropical Medicine*

AND

J. E. PURVIS, M.A., *University Lecturer in Chemistry and Physics in their application to Hygiene and Preventive Medicine, and Secretary to the State Medicine Syndicate*

T0372349

CANNED FOODS
IN RELATION TO HEALTH

CANNED FOODS
IN RELATION TO HEALTH
(*MILROY LECTURES* 1923)

BY

WILLIAM G. SAVAGE,
B.Sc., M.D. (Lond.), D.P.H.

County Medical Officer of Health, Somerset;
Examiner in State Medicine and Hygiene, London University;
Examiner in Public Health, University of Wales.

CAMBRIDGE
AT THE UNIVERSITY PRESS
1923

CAMBRIDGE
UNIVERSITY PRESS

University Printing House, Cambridge CB2 8BS, United Kingdom

Cambridge University Press is part of the University of Cambridge.

It furthers the University's mission by disseminating knowledge in the pursuit of education, learning and research at the highest international levels of excellence.

www.cambridge.org
Information on this title: www.cambridge.org/9781107494848

© Cambridge University Press 1923

This publication is in copyright. Subject to statutory exception and to the provisions of relevant collective licensing agreements, no reproduction of any part may take place without the written permission of Cambridge University Press.

First published 1923
First paperback edition 2015

A catalogue record for this publication is available from the British Library

ISBN 978-1-107-49484-8 Paperback

Cambridge University Press has no responsibility for the persistence or accuracy of URLs for external or third-party internet websites referred to in this publication, and does not guarantee that any content on such websites is, or will remain, accurate or appropriate.

PREFACE

THE book consists of the Milroy Lectures for 1923 as delivered in February and March before the Royal College of Physicians, London, with slight amplification in a few directions.

While available literature has been utilized I have mainly relied on a systematic and detailed laboratory study of canned foods upon which I have been engaged, with the help of other workers, during the last four years, and upon what may be termed field inquiries which I have made, dealing with methods of manufacture in this country, the United States of America and Canada and with the degree and methods of supervision exercised over their manufacture, importation and sale.

The literature on the subject is not considerable considering its importance, while it is very scattered and much of it not very accessible. For the convenience of workers a bibliography is included.

The aggregation of a large percentage of civilized populations in great centres has necessitated revision of the methods of food supply. In consequence a striking phenomenon of the present century is the ever increasing extent to which the food of the community is presented to them not in the fresh condition but preserved, so that they have made available the food of periods of plenty and from areas of abundance. So far as this relates to decomposable food it is entirely a modern phenomenon only possible through the application of scientific knowledge. Is this drastic change one to be encouraged whole heartedly or is it, like so many modern contrivances, fraught with its own menace and disadvantages which have to be eliminated or at least guarded against, before its benefits can be reaped ?

Of the many different methods of food preservation the procedure by which the food is preserved through being contained in hermetically sealed receptacles after treatment by heat is one which has increased by very rapid strides and the figures set out in the text show that the trade in canned goods is one of vast magnitude. The Great War caused an immense extension of their use and has supplied an object lesson—if one was needed—of the fact that canned foods have ceased to be a subsidiary means of supply and must be regarded as an essential source of food when large bodies of men or women have to be concentrated in a small area and subjected to conditions under which methods of transport are a primary consideration.

In view of their importance it is rather surprising that the matter has not received more general and detailed study from the Public Health point of view. In these Lectures I have attempted to give a comprehensive review, although of necessity somewhat condensed, of the whole subject of canned foods in their relationship to Public Health. The responsibility for any views expressed is entirely my own and these views do not, of necessity, reflect those of any Government Department with which I may have been associated.

Appendices I and II are two Reports by the author presented to the Canned Food Committee of the Food Investigation Board and included with their permission.

I am indebted to Dr Fitzgerald of the American Can Company for the illustrations on p. 126 and for permission to reproduce them.

W. G. S.

WESTON-SUPER-MARE.
October 1923.

CONTENTS

LECTURE I

SHORT HISTORICAL ACCOUNT OF THE CANNING INDUSTRY

THE introduction of the art of canning is due in large part to the stimulus of war, since it originated in the bounty of 12,000 francs offered by the French Government during the Napoleonic Wars for an improved method of preserving foods. The immediate object of the bounty was the reduction of food waste of Military and Naval stores.

Its wide extension in the United States of America was materially influenced by the demonstration of the utility and safety of foods so preserved during the American Civil War.

The French prize was ultimately awarded in 1810 to Nicholas Appert. His experiments continued from 1795 to 1810 and, although most of his earlier ones were failures, in the end success was achieved. His products were all packed in glass bottles. The food covered with water was placed in these bottles, these were corked and then heated in an open water bath, the length of time depending upon the character of the food. Although his procedure differs materially from practices now followed his principles were sound, and modern developments are largely advances in detail and in technique not involving new principles.

The commercial practice of canning dates from about 1820. The history of the industry is one of steady development. For example as regards the retainers used, glass was replaced by hand-made tins then by machine-made tins. The tins were first of the hole and cap variety requiring solder to seal; these in turn have been very generally replaced by the so-called "sanitary" or open top can in which no solder is used to fix on the lid. The latter type of can is quite modern and had its first extensive use in California in 1910.

In the same way there has been a gradual extension of the kinds of food canned until now almost every kind of food is found put up in tins. In the early stages of the industry local crops were bought up or were home grown on a small scale, if fruit or vegetables. Now it is recognized that the best results are obtained when the canner controls the crops or is his own farmer. Great attention is paid to the types of a fruit or vegetable which "can" best and after much selection these types only are cultivated specially for canning purposes. Some types of food have only been canned comparatively recently.

Thus while the canning of peas dates back to the beginnings of the industry, sardines were canned in 1834, and tomatoes in 1847, corn was only canned commercially after 1862. The first salmon cannery was established on the Sacramento river in 1864, on the Columbia river in 1866, in British Columbia in 1874 and in Alaska in 1882. The first patent for the manufacture of unsweetened condensed milk was granted to Borden, an American, in 1856 and was manufactured and sold by him in 1858. The Anglo-Swiss Condensed Milk Company built their first factory for sweetened Condensed Milk in Switzerland in 1866.

The development of the technical side of the industry has also been enormous and continuous. At first simple hand-worked factories were the rule. Before 1880 but little machinery was used in the industry but since that date its history has been the introduction of machine after machine to reduce labour and speed up production. Many of the machines now employed are of the most complicated and intricate construction. At the present time nearly all the stages are carried through by machinery and in a well equipped modern factory the food itself is comparatively little touched by hand. Each large factory contains thousands of pounds worth of machinery and the number of finished tins of a food turned out in a day may reach a hundred thousand or more. There are however many quite small factories with but few machines.

Material improvements have also been effected in the technical stages such as that of "processing" or sterilization. The open water bath has been replaced by jacketed retorts in which steam under pressure can act on the contained can, rotary retorts have been introduced to facilitate the penetration of the heat and improved methods of cooling afterwards have been adopted.

The general sanitary improvements in factories generally have also been reflected in canneries and I believe have taken place at an accelerated rate, while the reduction of wastage and the economical disposal of waste materials is now receiving serious consideration.

The last phase of progress has been the removal of the industry from one of mere empiricism to one built upon scientific foundations. This stage undoubtedly has lagged greatly and it is only during the last half dozen years or so that any serious and sustained endeavour has been made to try and explain, and so have power to control, the scientific principles involved, the causation of unsoundness and the basis of the precautions necessary to prevent loss from the contents becoming unfit.

Appert ascribed the preservation of the foods by his method to the exclusion of outside air, but naturally was ignorant of the scientific reason, while Gay Lussac, the distinguished French chemist appointed by his Government to investigate the cause of these foods keeping sound, reported that spoilage was the result of a series of oxidation changes which were prevented by the exclusion of the outside air. This view held the field until the development of bacteriology enabled a true explanation to be given. It is proposed in these lectures to submit the results of much exhaustive experimental work upon which I have been engaged, which it is hoped has carried our knowledge a stage further and thrown light upon some of the fundamental factors involved.

THE PRINCIPLES INVOLVED IN THE METHODS OF MANUFACTURE

It would occupy several lectures to give even an abridged account of the methods of preparation of the different varieties of canned foods. Fortunately such an account is not necessary to the scope of these lectures but it is essential to devote a little time to the principles involved which have a direct bearing upon the Public Health aspects of the subject.

The raw material. Outside the trade it is not generally realized how essential it is to obtain the right qualities of food for canning. This applies to nearly every kind of food canned. For example with sardines great care has to be taken to preserve the fish with an empty alimentary canal and they are usually kept alive in the weirs for 24 hours to free them from feed. Specially lean beasts alone are employed for meat canning and the use of the fattened Christmas ox would ruin the most careful meat canner owing to the unsightly over-fatty product. Equal care has to be taken with vegetables and fruit so much so that the most successful canners have become their own farmers and either grow or rigidly control their own supplies. Growing corn for canning must be watched almost daily so as to cut it when precisely ripe and soft enough. Freshness not only may affect the bacterial content but also the trade value of the finished product. Peas and beans for instance, stored if only for a few hours become less delicate and sweet. Special grades of fruit and vegetables are selected and grown specially for canning purposes.

Treatment at the factory before the food goes into the tin. The processes vary greatly according to the food packed and only a few which have a sanitary bearing can be mentioned. An important point is the continued introduction of machinery which diminishes handling. This markedly reduces the liability to bacterial contamination of the food while in the factory. The actual transfer of the food into the cans is frequently done by hand but otherwise there is often no handling at all.

A second point is that at some part of these stages the food often undergoes some heating. Sardines for example are distributed singly on trays by machinery and then cooked in single chambered steam heated ovens. Meat is partially cooked before filling into the cans. Many vegetables and fruit are "blanched" by hot water. Milk is pasteurized and often heated to temperatures above those ordinarily used in pasteurization.

These processes of preliminary heating are not, for the most part, devised to kill any bacteria present and they do not in any degree effect sterilization but they do kill out a good many organisms.

Steps to exclude air after closure of the tin. This is technically known as "exhausting" and from the sanitary point of view has two important advantages. It excludes air and it leaves a vacuum in the finished product. It will be shown later on that the exclusion of air is of primary importance in relation to spoilage while the methods of the Food inspectors to judge between sound and unsound tins are largely based upon the detection of this vacuum. Except for milk, and but little for sardines, all tinned foods should show, if sound, some vacuum within the tin. Apart from meat this is always obtained by the food being hot before the tin is hermetically closed. With some foods such as corn, peas or other vegetables a special process is not necessary as either the food is heated in the preparation or hot brine is added but with others the heating is obtained by passing the tins before closure in orderly sequence through boxes filled with steam. For meat the older practice was to pass through such an "exhaust box" but the plan now usually followed is to obtain the vacuum by the use of a vacuum sealing machine in which the air is sucked out by connection to an exhaust pump, the tins being sealed in the machine.

Addition of adjuvants. These are added to a good many foods, examples being tomato purée to herrings and sardines, olive oil or mustard sauce to sardines, syrup to most fruits, brine to many vegetables, meat jelly to meat, saccharose to milk. It is important that these should be free from living bacteria or moulds while they materially affect the potentialities for bacterial growth of the food.

The containers and the methods of closure. Both the quality of the container used and the efficiency of its hermetical closure are of immense technical importance. A bad quality of tin plate will cause great loss from pin-holing, action of the food (fruit especially) upon the metal and other defects resulting in spoilage. The most used type of can has an open top, the lid being fixed on by bending the edges of the top of the can and the flange of the lid by passing it through a double seamer machine. The joint so made should be air tight but usually requires some form of gasket (paper, rubber composition etc.) to be used to fill up the interstices to make it so. A leaky joint is a common cause of spoilage.

"Processing." This is a stage of primary importance in relation to bacterial soundness and is only omitted for sweetened condensed milk where the sugar added is relied upon to maintain soundness. It is the technical term applied in the trade to the final heating given to the product in the can after it has been hermetically sealed and is designed to render the product safe from subsequent bacterial decomposition. It is supposed to sterilize the product, i.e. to render it free from living bacteria but it will be shown in Lecture 2 that this object is only attained in a proportion of cases. It is by no means the simple problem it is often supposed to be of the application of a definite degree of heat for a given time with the resultant of a sterile product. The factors governing its efficiency are of extreme complexity and are discussed in some detail in Appendix No. 1.

The tins are cooled directly after heating and should be incubated and examined after storage to see if they remain sound.

From these brief notes it is evident that while the actual principles involved are few and definite the technical difficulties are numerous and troublesome. It is only after a long pupillage that the industry has been established on its present sound commercial basis.

GROWTH AND EXTENT OF THE INDUSTRY

It is a matter of considerable difficulty to obtain full information as to the amount of canned foods prepared in the world and as to the amount consumed in this country. The Board of Trade tables of imports of canned foods are no guide to the amount of imported canned foods consumed because a material proportion of the goods so scheduled are re-exported without being further dealt with in this country. The most useful guide to the amount of imported canned foods consumed is obtained from the following table, abstracted from the Board of Trade returns, and which shows the quantities retained in this country. It is not an absolute index of the imported tinned food consumed in the particular year indicated because there are likely to be some variations in the stocks held in wholesalers' and retailers' hands at the beginning and at the end of the year but the correction cannot be large and does not affect the essential accuracy of the figures.

TABLE I

Total quantities of Foreign and Colonial canned foods retained in the United Kingdom. (Figures in cwts.)

Canned Food	Year 1913	Year 1920	Year 1921
Beef (including tongues)	not available	93,176	337,429
Mutton (including tongues) ...	not available	130,861	48,261
Meat (not otherwise specified) ...	not available	63,147	64,849
Marine products:			
Herrings	—[1]	12,633	8,192
Sardines	171,545[3]	—[2]	49,146
Salmon	525,850	781,819	514,851
Lobsters	12,336	14,435	26,277
Other sorts	51,370	42,861	54,822
Fruit (canned and bottled) ...	852,019	1,275,853	1,319,572
Vegetables (canned and bottled)[4]...	462,330	446,243	447,213
Milk: unsweetened	39,065	89,050	558,625
„ sweetened, whole ...	465,287	1,226,303	670,784
„ „ separated or skimmed ...	719,696	462,725	871,924

No figures are available as to the extent to which canned foods are manufactured in this country. The following table shows that a certain quantity is exported.

TABLE II

Exports of canned foods manufactured in the United Kingdom. (Figures in cwts.)

Canned food	Year 1920	Year 1921
Meats	10,564	12,550
Marine products: herrings	189,018	66,571
„ „ other sorts	27,456	7,762
Fruit (canned and bottled) ...	2,888	2,308
Vegetables (canned and bottled) ...	3,090	2,825
Milk: unsweetened	5,116	13,569
„ sweetened, whole	53,576	22,727
„ „ separated or skimmed	861	—

[1] Included in "other sorts" in 1913.
[2] Re-exports in excess of imports.   [3] Includes "Brisling" in 1913.
[4] Tomatoes are included as vegetables.

It is of interest to follow out the places of manufacture of these imports. This cannot be given for the net imports but it is available for the year 1920 for the total imports, i.e. inclusive of the canned foods which are not retained but are exported again. These figures however are more valuable when it is merely a question of indicating the countries of manufacture. The following tables are abstracted from Vol. II, Table I, of the Board of Trade Annual Statement.

TABLE III

Imports of canned meats: year 1920. (*Figures in cwts.*)

Source	Beef	Mutton	Rabbit	Meat not other-wise specified
United States of America	58,069	2,642	—	45,573
South America	381,858	10,258	—	8,903
Other foreign countries...	29,563	327	4	4,145
Australia	161,658	96,393	28,978	3,212
New Zealand	64,404	30,796	16,772	668
Canada	10,857	506	} 43	8,646
Other British possessions	6,952	3,412		937
Total	713,361	144,334	45,797	72,084

TABLE IV

Imports of canned marine products: year 1920. (*Figures in cwts.*)

Source	Herrings	Sardines	Salmon	Lobster	Other sorts
Norway	14,652	—	—	—	43,100
France...	465	17,358	—	29	3,510
Portugal	—	47,607	—	—	—
U.S.A....	—	445	325,455	—	9,903
Japan	—	—	354,248	—	2,657
Canada	—	—	156,638	23,439	—
Other British posses-sions	—	—	306	1,547	36,869
Other foreign countries	344	5,178	13,297	20	11,341
Total	15,461	70,588	849,944	25,035	107,380

TABLE V

Condensed milk and fruit imports: year 1920. (*Figures in cwts.*)

Source	Unsweetened	Sweetened (whole)	Sweetened (separated or skimmed)	Fruit (canned and bottled)
Norway	2,887	3,114	2,483	—[1]
Denmark	189	16,038	34,883	—[1]
Netherlands	425	60,444	419,308	19,649
France	257	30,262	25	19,892
Switzerland	3,116	22,667	—	—[1]
U.S.A.	246,735	829,830	4,145	732,986
Other Foreign Countries	2,061	40,986	1,569	187,616[2]
Straits Settlements and Dependencies ...	0	6,841	} 2,171	164,626
Australia	0	12,298		89,460
New Zealand	0	7,125		—[3]
Canada...	13,361	210,128		100,366
Other British Possessions	0	1,122		5,387

The following figures give a good idea of the extension of the industry in U.S.A. but figures for the last few years are not available.

TABLE VI[4]

Product	Figures per	1899	1904	1909	1914	1917
Tomatoes	million cases	8·7	9·4	12·9	16·2	15·1
Vegetables (excluding tomatoes)	,,	10·6	20·2	19·8	32·9	38·6
Fruit (excluding tomatoes)	,,	4·5	4·6	5·5	9·4	15·3
Marine products ...	million lbs.	117·2	207·0	235·4	—	—
Meats	,,	112·4	—	121·4	—	—
Sweetened condensed milk...	,,	} 186·9	198·3	214·5	—	—
Unsweetened condensed milk ...	,,		110·1	280·3	—	—

[1] Included with "Other Foreign Countries."
[2] Includes 116,077 cwts. imported from Spain.
[3] Included with "Other British Possessions."
[4] Compiled from *Report of the Federal Trade Commission on Canned Foods*, May 1918, Washington, U.S.A., and *U.S.A. Department of Agriculture Bulletin*, No. 195, "Methods followed in the Commercial Canning of Foods," Washington, 1915.

Corn, peas and tomatoes are typical U.S.A. canned products and the following figures from reports of the National Canners Association are of interest as showing the increase in the quantities canned. The tomato figures do not correspond exactly with those in the last table, probably due to the inclusion of tomato purée in one case and not in the other.

Table VII

Figures per million cases.

Year	Corn	Peas	Tomatoes
1908	6·8	5·6	11·5
1909	5·8	5·0	11·0
1910	10·0	4·4	9·2
1911	14·3	4·5	9·7
1912	13·1	7·0	14·0
1913	7·3	8·8	14·2
1914	9·8	8·8	15·2
1915	10·1	9·3	8·5
1916	9·1	6·7	13·1
1917	10·8	9·8	15·1
1918	11·7	11·0	15·9
1919	13·6	8·7	10·8
1920	15·0	12·3	11·4

The only figures available to me showing the amount of canned foods manufactured in the country are for milk and for the year 1919 only. The Interdepartmental Committee Report on Condensed Milk gives the following figures.

Skimmed sweetened condensed milk   127,942 cwts.
Full cream   „   „   „   1,199,705 cwts.
Unsweetened condensed milk   84,028 cwts.

Although the figures are incomplete they show clearly how very large is the canned food industry and how material a part it contributes to the food supply of this country. While the importations of some classes of foods do not appear to be extending it seems generally true that not only is an increasing variety of foods being canned but that more and more of each kind is canned. The 1918 U.S.A. Report on Canned Foods states that the Census of 1914 showed 4220 canning establishments in that country with 88,069 persons engaged.

The general increase in the industry year by year suggests that we cannot regard the figures reached as the maximum and that we shall have to look forward to yet further developments in the number of foods canned with a still larger output of this type of preserved food.

It will be convenient here to consider to what extent this industry is likely to extend in Great Britain. Since this country is one which has to import a material proportion of its food supply it is obvious that it will not develop into a great canning centre. There are however certain foods which do offer scope for canning. Of these fish is the most important, since certain species of fish are at times considerably more abundant than can be disposed of in their fresh condition. A certain amount of fish is canned in this country but the difficulties of establishing the business on a commercial footing are many and considerable.

Sprats and herrings are fish which have received careful consideration as possibly suitable to "can" in this country. An incomplete account of the British Canned Fish Industry, with some discussion on the possibility of its extension, has recently been published by Professor Johnstone[1] (1921). As he there points out at no place on the British coasts could a cannery depend on local supplies of freshly-caught fish throughout the year. The heavy cost of land transport makes it impracticable to transport fish to a fixed cannery, say on the East Coast, from other fishery ports in England where the fish might be at any one time plentiful. There is no doubt that one, and probably the main, difficulty is the fact that the season of abundance at

[1] The references are given in the bibliography at the end.

any one part of the British coast is a very short one and therefore a fish canning factory would only be running for a very short period. This period could be lengthened a little by changing over and canning more than one kind of fish but this introduces complications which add to the cost. The possibility of temporarily preserving superfluous fish in brine or by other means and so evening and spreading out the canning period has been considered, but the experimental work done, discussed by Johnstone (*loc. cit.*), is not encouraging.

Seasonal difficulties occur however in other countries and have been overcome. For example the flourishing sardine canning industry which centres round Eastport (Maine State, U.S.A.) has to contend with a marked seasonal fluctuation.

There is also a possible method of dealing with the problem of abundance of fish for several weeks at different centres on the British coast which might be worth consideration. If the fish cannot be conveyed profitably to the cannery the cannery might go to the fish. In salmon canning the most recent type of fish cannery is a vessel which is floated to a point near the fishing grounds. It is possible to fit up a cannery on a vessel and it might be feasible to move it to the places of fish abundance and can there until the supply is exhausted.

Of other products, a considerable amount of sweetened and some unsweetened condensed milk is prepared in this country and is a valuable means for dealing with surplus spring and summer supplies of milk. In addition a good deal of made up meat products are put up in glass or metal retainers and a certain amount of fruit is bottled or canned.

Speaking generally, however, the volume of food preserved by canning or bottling in this country is inconsiderable compared with the total amount so preserved.

SUPERVISION EXERCISED OVER
CANNED FOODS

Apart from the magnitude of the industry there are special reasons why this class of foods needs supervision in addition to that provided under the ordinary regulations controlling food generally. Of these reasons the most important is that they are mostly made up products and consequently the use of unsound constituents is less easily detected than if the whole product alone was available. This can best be brought out by a few examples. It is well known that the detection of diseased conditions in meat is facilitated by an examination of the viscera, indeed such detection may be impossible without. The musculature of highly diseased animals may show no obtrusive signs although bacterially infective, the whole of the gross lesions being concentrated in the viscera and other internal organs. In canned meat only the carcase is used and no one can reliably detect from the contents of a tin whether the animal from which it was derived was healthy or not. Apart from bacteriological examination of the milk from each individual tin, and that may be ineffective due to sterilization, there is no means of ascertaining if it came from diseased cows, unless the milk was markedly altered in consistency. Another reason for special supervision is the difficulty of detecting the use of damaged products in a state of incipient putrefaction. This more particularly applies to fish. The "processing" given may result in a sterile product but not free from the products of putrefaction or other bacterial change and the heat changes may so alter the product that it is a matter of the greatest difficulty to determine the precise condition as regards the soundness of the product as canned.

It will be shown in Lecture III that it is not very uncommon for a meat or fish product to retain, with virulence unimpaired, the toxins of the Salmonella group and without any possibility of further detection by any physical examination of the contents or of the outside of the retainer.

The possibility of the use of insufficiently cleaned products is one which specially applies to fruit and vegetables. Tomatoes for example are often heavily earth contaminated and demand the most thorough washing. All earth laden fruit may convey the spores of *B. botulinus* and such canned products may show no defects externally and comparatively little when opened and examined.

Lastly it must be borne in mind that there are preserved foods which may and often are kept for prolonged periods. During that time the possibility of prejudicial changes taking place in the contents or the addition of poisonous bodies such as tin from the retainers must not be overlooked.

For these various reasons it is obvious that some special supervision is necessary and at different stages in the passage of these foods from the raw product to the consumer.

SUPERVISION AT THE SOURCE

While canned foods are made in many parts of the world the largest production is in the United States of America and special attention is directed here to the conditions in that country. I am not in possession of the methods of supervision at the source in other countries although I have studied them at first hand to some extent in Canada. As regards this country no special supervision is exercised. The manufacturers of canned food products are liable to inspection under the Public Health Laws and regulations in the same way as other food producers but there is no special code of regulations to conform to and no inspectorial staff set apart to supervise canned food products. A certain amount of canned food of various kinds is made in this country and in view of the special needs for supervision set out above it would certainly seem desirable that more attention should be devoted to their preparation. It is not enough to rely upon the high standards which manufacturers in this country have set and, so far as I have been able to judge, reach.

It will I think be of interest to give a short account of methods in the United States of America since so much is imported from that country.

Official supervision in the United States of America. This is complicated because there are two series of laws —those enforced by the Federal Government and those by the individual States. The Federal Laws which apply are the Food and Drugs Act 1906, and the Meat Inspection Act 1906.

The Food and Drugs Act 1906 is a comprehensive Act which is enforced by the Bureau of Chemistry. It forbids the importation, the shipment in interstate or foreign commerce, or the manufacture and sale in any part of the United States of adulterated or misbranded foods or drugs. Under it a series of Regulations has been promulgated from time to time which constitute an extensive mass of enactments. Unlike the powers in the Meat Inspection Act it does not give authority for the continuous maintenance of inspectors in all establishments manufacturing food products and nothing of this sort can be attempted. Under it, however, the Bureau does carry out a good deal of systematic investigation of plants where foods and drugs shipped in interstate commerce are made. The procedures adopted to maintain a high standard of food product are, in general, similar to those employed in this country and are the collection and analysis of samples of the product suspected of being in violation of the Act. If the results warrant further action, legal proceedings are taken.

It will be noted that the Federal supervision is exercised only over foods and drugs passing from one State to another or shipped out of the country but has no control over products made and sold within the confines of a single State. Circular 137 of the Bureau of Chemistry states that most of the States have food and drug laws similar in many respects to the Federal Act and designed to afford the same protection.

The Meat Inspection Act of 1906 and the supplementary legislation in the tariff Act of 1913 gives extensive powers in regard to the Federal inspection of meat and meat products. The 1906 Act applies to the slaughtering, packing, rendering and meat-preparing in establishments which sell or ship their products in whole or in part in interstate or foreign commerce. It does not apply to establishments which only sell their products within the confines of a single State.

This inspection is under the Bureau of Animal Industry and I am indebted to Dr J. R. Mohler, Chief of the Bureau, for the following particulars of their working.

"Only meats which have been 'Inspected and Passed' and so marked and which are handled in accordance with the regulations may be admitted into establishments where meats are canned for export. All meats are subject to identification and inspection at the time of admission and are reinspected from time to time to insure that only those which remain sound and wholesome and are handled in a sanitary manner are utilized for human food.

All establishments which "can" export meats are required to have Federal inspection as prescribed by law and the regulations. These establishments are under the immediate supervision of Federal inspectors who personally perform the inspections and see that there is due and satisfactory compliance with the regulations governing the sanitation of establishments and equipment, the cleanly handling of meats throughout, including storage, packing, processing, labelling, etc.

The Federal meat inspection service has seven laboratories located at advantageous centres throughout the United States for the purpose of maintaining laboratory supervision over the operations of establishments where meats are prepared and canned. The laboratory inspection of canned meats is directly connected with the inspection within the establishments. It begins with sampling all materials used in the preparation, curing and handling of meats, and includes examination of all curing substances, spices, condiments, etc. Every ingredient and all substances and materials used are subject to laboratory examination. The water supplies of establishments are examined at regular intervals to insure purity and potability. Samples of the finished canned meats are also examined from time to time to insure wholesomeness, proper sterilization and processing, correctness of the statement of net weight and correctness of labelling."

Undoubtedly the Federal Meat Inspection service is one of the most (if not the most) complete systems of meat inspection in the world. Some 2500 employees, including veterinary, laboratory, and lay Inspectors, are continuously engaged in this work. Dr Mohler adds:

"No meats are permitted to be exported unless the meats or containers thereof bear marks of Federal inspection and to all of the principal foreign countries they are accompanied by export certificates issued by the Secretary of Agriculture and countersigned by the inspector showing the meats to be from animals that were free from disease, and that they have been inspected and passed as sound and wholesome as provided by the law and regulations."

I have had some personal experience of this work in the stockyards of Chicago and was impressed with the careful control exercised and with the capacity of the Officers in charge of this very important branch of public health.

While the supervision over meat is rigid, special Federal supervision does not appear to be exercised over fish and other products, but they come under the ordinary laws. The valuable *Bulletin* (No. 908) issued in 1921 on the Maine sardine industry originated out of examinations of sardines under the Federal Food and Drugs Acts, and no special sanitary regulations are mentioned.

Supervision by the trade. While trade Associations exist in many parts of the world they are mainly established for purely trade purposes, including the regulation of prices. The National Canners Association in U.S.A. has, however, done valuable work in connection with the improvement of the food products of their members along Public Health lines and in elucidating technical problems so that the following brief account of its activities will be of interest.

National Canners Association inspections. This Association has organized a system of inspection for the benefit of their constituents. The scheme is organized from the Headquarters of the Association in Washington, but is developed mainly on divisional or local lines. The Association has a separate Inspection service under the direction of a National Director of Inspection with an Advisory Board composed of the National Director and the directors of inspection of the several districts. The canning areas are marked out into territories which may or may not be coterminous with States. Each territory has its own staff of Directors with a number of Inspectors, and in some cases with a local laboratory and staff. The general trend of the Inspection is to secure

(*a*) That each factory shall be sanitary in construction and particularly as regards its working.

(*b*) That good quality food only shall be used.

(*c*) That the grading shall be an accurate description and that cans shall be filled and contain a proper proportion of the food.

The Inspectors and Directors not only inspect but give advice as regards the technical conduct of the operations.

The cost of the whole scheme is borne by the canners who join the Association and is assessed at a charge per case which varies from 1·25 to 2 cents per case.

In their byelaws stress is laid upon the qualifications required to become a member of the Association. These include that the firms which are members must conduct their plants in a sanitary manner and use only wholesome raw products, and sterilized by the use of heat alone and that no chemicals for preservative purposes may be used. Members adversely reported upon in this connection are liable to be expelled from membership.

The advantages to the canner are threefold:

1. If everything is satisfactory certificates are issued, attached to each case, that the goods have been inspected and packed under supervision. Canned goods with this

certificate fetch a higher price and this makes it worth the canner's while to have them.

2. It helps to bring up the whole quality of the particular branch of canned goods packed and tends to prevent the sanitary packer who spends money on sanitary premises from being prejudiced by the competition of those packers who are able to pack cheaper because they are less sanitary.

3. He obtains the benefit of the advice and practical help of the scientific staff of the N.C.A. How valuable this help should be, and I believe is, is clear from a study of the admirable technical bulletins issued by the Association.

During my visit to the United States in 1919 I had numerous opportunities of studying the work of this Association and of visiting factories run by members of it, and also of those not members. I was very favourably impressed with the influence it was exerting to improve the conditions under which the industry was carried on, while it was equally evident that the scientific studies on the different technical problems connected with canning were gradually removing the procedure from an empirical to a scientific basis.

There are other Canning Associations in America, some of which are purely local, others only an association of packers of one particular commodity. I am not aware that any of these carry out any inspection work on the lines of the National Association, but they all lay stress upon their educational activities. How far any of these other trade associations are concerned in the question of the prices at which they are to sell their commodities I have no means of judging. As regards the National Canners Association their secretary, in a personal communication, lays stress upon the fact that they are in no way concerned in the question of prices nor do they exert any influence upon this factor.

CONTROL EXERCISED OVER CANNED FOODS AT
THE PORTS OF ENTRY

The considerable powers possessed by Port and other Dock-side Authorities are derived from the Unsound Food Regulations 1908.

Article IV gives the Medical Officer of Health power to examine any article of food which has been landed within the district and, if necessary, before it has been landed. If the tinned food or other article examined is found to be unsound or unwholesome or unfit for human food the article may be seized and, after compliance with certain requirements, destroyed. Alternately he may serve a written notice requiring that the articles of food shall not be removed without permission from the place of examination, or from any other place specified in the notice, until the article of food has been examined by a Justice.

In practice powers of detention of a consignment are more used than seizure since the latter involves the carrying away of the articles. As worked this section is read as if it permitted the detention of the whole of a consignment when it has been ascertained that a certain proportion of the tins composing it are unsound. A printed notice is served requiring the detention of the whole batch pending its detailed examination.

Article VIII gives powers of sampling. It also provides, pending the examination of such a sample, that the person in charge of the consignment shall not distribute it but afford facilities for its detailed examination within a reasonable period by the M.O.H. or his assistants.

While these powers are useful they do not give any very extensive control over imported canned foods.

This will be clearer if a short description is given as to what happens in actual practice in such a large port as London. At least three different procedures may be followed with a ship containing consignments of canned foods.

It may go direct to one of the widely scattered docks in London and discharge its cargo there. In this case the responsibility for its examination rests with the Port of London Sanitary Authority. It may go direct to a wharfside and discharge its cargo directly on to the wharf and the onus of being satisfied as to the satisfactory condition of the consignment is then on the Local Authority in whose area the wharf is situated. In the third place it may discharge its canned food consignment by barge from the ship in the river or from within the dock. In either case the responsibility for the purity of the food is on the Authority in whose area the wharf is situated.

In practice a considerable amount of intercommunication takes place between the different London Riverside Sanitary Authorities concerned and the Port of London Sanitary Authority under a series of joint orders.

These differences are of practical importance because the main source of information of the Local Authority is from the Bills of Lading (Bill A). When the ship directly discharges at dock side or along a wharf these are available but they are not when the goods are discharged by barge without coming alongside. In the latter event it is possible for a considerable parcel of canned goods to be brought into the area of a Riverside Authority without any official information being received, and they would have to rely upon the goods being noted by the Food Inspector in his routine and special visits to the wharfs and warehouses.

There is no obligation on the part of any importer to notify the Port or Local Sanitary Authority of the fact that goods are being landed.

One indirect source of information is however available, and is of some utility. The Port Authorities and H.M. Customs usually work in co-operation, and it is the practice of the latter to notify the former of all defective consignments of canned goods which appear to them to require examination.

Another source of information which is valuable and considerably utilized is the results of examinations of canned goods made by and for the trade. It is a common, but by no means an invariable, practice for importers to buy this type of food on the basis of a ten per cent. or other percentage examination. On the results of such an examination an allowance is made for defective tins.

These examinations are made by persons employed by the wharf owners, who usually act as agents in this matter, and whose staff, although working on rule of thumb lines, obtain a high degree of expertness in the work. Their rejections are not, as I have shown in several special reports, accurate as regards tins with sound and unsound contents, but they are accurate as regards sound and unsound tins. In effect their examination results in the rejection of all tins which are imperfect in any way and which in fact are tins which the wholesale buyer would reject as unsound and liable to be thrown back on his hands by the retail buyer.

While the results of these examinations generally do come to the notice of the Inspectors of the Port or Local Sanitary Authorities there are no powers to demand this information and no obligation to supply it.

In practice if the Food Inspector finds the proportion of rejects to be a high one, and the definition of "high" varies in the different ports and to a certain extent with the class of food canned, he suggests the need for a complete examination of the whole consignment which he generally supervises but rarely carries out himself. As already explained the whole consignment is detained at the wharf pending such an examination, but there does not appear to be any legal authority for such detention. It is more a matter of good will and expediency.

It is true Section IV gives powers of detention but this is only when, after examination, the Medical Officer of Health is of opinion that a particular article of food is unsound or unwholesome or unfit for human food. It is at least very doubtful whether this gives legal sanction for the detention of a consignment which is a mixture of good and bad tins. He has not examined all the tins and the powers of detention only apply to a specific article *after* it has been examined.

The working of the Regulations is an interesting illustration of a feature common in Public Health administration, i.e. of a defective legal machinery which by the exercise of common sense and good will is yet in practice a valuable workable scheme of control. To the outsider it does, however, exhibit many flaws and possibilities of complete lack of control.

There is, for example, no obligation at all on a Port or Local Sanitary Authority to examine consignments of canned foods. There may be wide differences of procedure and complete lack of uniformity. One Authority may be lax in inspection work and greatly understaffed and become known in the trade as a suitable depository for poor quality canned goods. There appears to be nothing to prevent a low grade and defective parcel of canned food from being landed by barge on to a wharf, never coming to the official or actual cognizance of the Local Authority Officers, not being examined at all by anyone at the wharf and then being distributed through the country. As the Port and Local Sanitary Authorities are now staffed it is not possible for them themselves to examine more than a small percentage of the tins which come into the area of their Authority.

It would certainly seem desirable that the owners of all canned goods admitted into this country should be compelled to supply information of the consignment giving the source, nature of food packed, and the quantity. This information has to be supplied to the Customs Authority by the shipowners and with very little trouble could be sent also to the Riverside Sanitary Authority concerned.

It is desirable that the results of the trade examinations should be notified to the Port and Local Sanitary Riverside Authority, but it is hardly reasonable to suggest a legal compulsion since after all it is done solely for trade purposes, and the obvious retort of the trade would be that if the Local Authority want this information they have powers of examination and let them come and do their own work. This therefore must remain a matter of good will, while if it was pressed it would possibly become the practice to sell the goods without any examination at all.

Definite legal powers to detain a suspected consignment pending sorting out of the sound from the unsound are required.

Supervision after distribution. There are no regulations in this country dealing specially with the supervision of canned foods or any official documents setting out the criteria which should govern their condemnation. They can be, and are, dealt with under the laws which govern foods generally. If, for example, they are found unfit they can be seized, condemned by a magistrate and, if thought fit, legal action taken against the vendor.

The Health Officers of Local Authorities, which are not also Riverside Authorities, are not, in my experience, well versed in the special technical points which affect judgment of canned foods. There is need for the diffusion of more expert information as to the criteria upon which to judge an unopened tin and in regard to the information which such an examination can yield as to the character and wholesomeness of its contents.

THE VALUE AND LIMITATIONS OF THE
CONTROL EXERCISED

It will be appreciated that one way and another canned foods receive a good deal of supervision. In this country the most important line of defence is the work done at the Ports of entry. It is therefore of importance to consider critically its reliability and value.

In the first place it is evident from the descriptions given that while a good deal of the canned food imported into this country does not receive systematic inspection the supervision given is a valuable check upon the importation of consignments of unsound canned food. It has not yet been considered as to how far the actual inspection methods practised in this country are satisfactory and reliable. If perfect they should on the one hand be capable of eliminating every tin the contents of which contained harmful bacteria, were decomposed, or contained metals in poisonous amount or were otherwise prejudicial, while on the other hand they should enable every tin with sound contents to be passed and so prevent the wastage of valuable food.

It may be said at once that they are very far from yielding results approaching these desiderata. They are inadequate to detect the presence of harmful bacteria or their toxins when these bacilli do not produce decomposition or fermentative changes; they are unable to detect the presence of chemical poisons from an examination of the unopened tin. Thus they fail, and must fail with our present knowledge, to detect the really dangerous tins and any claim of this sort must be abandoned though it is sometimes advanced. It has however been claimed for the methods of examination practised that they do differentiate between the tin with undecomposed sound contents and the one in which the food has begun to break down and decompose.

The value of any such claim can only be judged by comparative investigation and critical study of the contents of passed and rejected tins. This has been specially investigated by me and the results are contained in a series of reports issued by the Food Investigation Board (see Bibliography). It will only be possible here to draw attention to the general results obtained.

It may be mentioned that the methods of examination employed strikingly resemble those used by a doctor for the physical examination of the human chest and include inspection, palpation, percussion and auscultation in the form of shake sound, etc. All are employed for meat and fish and most of them for other varieties of canned foods, but the stress laid upon the different tests is materially different for the different classes of foods. For example with meat the percussion note is of primary significance while with fruit, consisting as it does of a mixture of solids and liquids this note is of very little utility.

The following table gives in a very condensed form the results of the examinations carried out by my colleagues and myself.

TABLE VIII

Product	Number of samples examined			Number in which judgment of Food Inspector correct			Percentage in which judgment correct		
	Passed	Rejected	Total	Passed	Rejected	Total	Passed	Rejected	Total
Meat	16	57	73	15	15	30	94	26	41
Salmon ...	11	44	55	11	25	36	100	57	65·5
Sardines ...	6	25	31	5	11	16	83	44	51
Herrings ...	5	14	19	5	8	13	100	57	68
Crustacea ...	1	43	44	0	32	32	0	74	73
Sweetened condensed milk	1	44	45	0	39	39	0	89	87
Unsweetened condensed milk	6	51	57	5	47	52	83	92	91
Fruit	8	99	107	8	88	96	100	89	90
Total ...	54	377	431	49	265	314	91	70	73

Note to table. The crustacea comprise crab, lobster and crayfish. The figures only relate to suspected samples which were examined and rejected or passed by the Food Inspectors. The 54 tins which were passed by the Food Inspectors were all tins which were rejected as defective by the Trade Examiners. The correctness of the judgment given was obtained after a very full examination of the contents, i.e. physical appearance and characters when opened, full detailed bacteriological examination and chemical analysis.

While the table is interesting the crude figures cannot be utilized to compare the reliability of the methods for one product as against another, the sampling not being comparable. For some of the foods a special selection of doubtful and difficult tins was made. For a detailed discussion of the value and difficulties of the examination the different reports must be consulted.

What the table does bring out very clearly is that a very considerable number of tins with sound contents is rejected by the present methods. The subject is complicated and involves the discussion of physical laws, but it may be said here that while certain defects such for example as a "blown" tin are definitely associated with decomposition changes, other physical conditions such as an abnormal shake sound, or a "springy" condition of the metal container may be due to many causes only some of which are associated with conditions which render the contents unsound.

While something can be done to reduce the discrepancy between rejections and condition of contents the differences are largely beyond control unless improved methods of examination can be devised. The present methods of examination very rarely result in the passing of a tin the contents of which are decomposed but they do result in the rejection of large numbers of samples which are perfectly good. For some foods the percentage of sound samples condemned is not high enough to matter, but with other foods, such as meat and fish, there is a discrepancy which in practice leads to the loss of a considerable quantity of sound food. It is possible to reduce this wastage by appropriate means including the extension of laboratory facilities for examination and a closer co-ordination between laboratory examinations and the work of the Medical Officers of Health and their Food Inspectors.

CERTAIN SPECIAL POINTS RELATING TO INFORMATION ON THE TINS

In connection with the supervision and control of canned foods there are certain points which crop up and which are of great practical importance.

Labelling. In connection with the elucidation of outbreaks of food poisoning and for other purposes it is sometimes desirable to trace the whole of a particular consignment. One obstacle to this course is the unsatisfactory position as regards labelling. A good deal of canned food, and that often of lower grade, reaches this country unlabelled and is so purchased. Such a consignment may be all purchased by one firm and then divided up and sold to several firms. Each firm then puts on its own fancy label and particular designation, sometimes without any real guarantee as to the quality and purity of the contents. In other words the same pack of canned food may be vended under several quite different labels and be difficult to trace.

The converse may occur and be equally unsatisfactory. A firm in this country by lavish advertisement may acquire a reputation for a particular brand. It may be, for example, a particular brand of salmon which it buys unlabelled and then labels with its own fancy title. Its next purchase may be the same type of fish but may not be of the same quality or even from the same factory. It gets exactly the same label and may be sold side by side with the other. In other words the same label may cover different qualities of contents and packed at very different times or on the other hand one pack of canned food may be vended under several different labels.

Many canners do adopt a coding system which enables them to identify each can with the batch with which it was processed. This is valuable to the canner from the commercial point of view but it is a private system and is not available to either the Local Public Health or Central Health Authority who may wish to stop a whole consignment, one tin of which for example has caused an outbreak of botulism.

The actual source and local place of canning of the product should be stamped on the tin to facilitate identification. This need not be in full, but sufficient for identification through the Ministry of Health or other central authority.

Absence of date of canning. Considerable controversy has taken place over the question of the desirability of requiring the date of canning to be indicated on the tins. Many Public Health authorities have advocated this as desirable while the trade as a whole takes strong exception to any such requirement. I have discussed this matter with large scale canners in U.S.A. and heard their side of the question. Summed up their main contention is that it is unnecessary and misleading. If an article is canned properly then it is sterile and will keep indefinitely and is therefore just as good years hence. To enforce a date stamp would mean in practice that the public, being uneducated as to the keeping qualities of canned goods, would demand those only recently canned, and goods perfectly sound but not recently made would be rejected and thrown back upon the producers. This in effect would mean an increase in the price of canned goods to cover the loss. They also refer to the fact well known in the trade that certain canned foods, for example sardines, improve with age and that a well matured tin is preferable to a freshly canned one.

The argument is specious but depends upon two considerations for its validity. One is that the public is not educable, the other that canned goods do not deteriorate with time.

As regards the first point I do not think the public will trouble itself at all about the matter so long as the contents are good. If the contents after opening are found unsound, the purchaser would doubtless regard the fact that the tin was an old one as an aggravation of the matter, but I think he would be justified and that does not touch the argument. It is of interest and significance that during the war one requirement of the British Government, at least for some canned goods purchased, was that the date of preparation should be stamped on the tin, and I am unaware of any inconvenience or loss resulting from the practice.

Dealing with the second point it will be shown in the next lecture that canned foods cannot be regarded as sterile foods and that in many foods changes in consequence do result with time. There is considerable evidence that the "maturation" changes which slowly result in some canned foods are largely due to bacterial activities. These may or may not be beneficial or at least harmless, but we do not know. We are certainly not in a position to affirm that the contents of a several years old tin of canned food are just as good as the contents of a recently canned tin. There is no evidence either way, but dating the goods may help in obtaining it. Further in certain directions there is definite evidence that inimical changes do result from prolonged storage. For instance condensed milk, especially the sweetened type, definitely and markedly deteriorates with time, particularly at high temperatures. The solution of tin is directly influenced by the time factor. In very old tins it is possible for a large amount of tin to be dissolved by foods, such as fruits and fish, which act upon the container. The food may become actively poisonous (see Lecture III).

Also we have to realize that the vitamin content of

canned foods is influenced by time, and while the freshly made canned food may retain the greater part of its original content in vitamins storage will diminish and in time remove them.

While therefore it may be true that for some foods age does not prejudicially interfere with their quality it is not generally true, and a strong case can be made out for requiring that the date of preparation should be stamped on all tins of canned food made in or imported into this country.

Not only should the date be stamped but some code mark, disclosed to the Ministry of Health, whereby the tin can be traced back to the actual canning factory. If the canned foods are perfectly wholesome the trade has nothing to fear from such a requirement.

Repainting and touching up of damaged canned goods. This seems not uncommon as in connection with my studies at the Ports of entry I have several times come across the practice. A consignment is damaged by salt water, by labels being put on too wet etc., and a large proportion of the cans become rusty and unsightly. The labels are scraped off, the paint washed off, the tins examined and those which do not show rust holes are repainted and relabelled "as good as new." The practice is not desirable without disclosure to the Health authority since it is probable that many pin point leaks from rusting will be left and it will be shown in Lecture II that this air admission is a serious matter as regards spoilage. Incubation of the tins for some time before release seems desirable.

Standards as to chemical composition. Canned foods have come to stay and ultimately a good deal more attention will have to be paid to this question. In any case it should be obligatory for the net weight of the contents to be clearly marked on the tin or label. At the present time the only chemical standards of pressing importance are in regard to condensed milks. For both sweetened and unsweetened condensed milk there exists great variations as regards the degree of concentration of both and of the percentage of sugar for the sweetened variety. It should not, for example, be left to the public to try and discriminate between an unsweetened milk concentrated from double the volume of milk and one concentrated threefold. Obviously the two are of very unequal nutritive value. This aspect of the subject has been fully dealt with by Dr Coutts in 1911, but legal standards still lag in the making although in Section 8 of the Milk and Dairies (Amendment) Act 1922 powers are now available for this purpose[1].

As regards one variety—condensed machine skimmed milk—it is difficult to see any need for it at all. So long as it is obtainable and the cheapest condensed milk available, so long will the less discriminating and poorer sections of the community, harassed by their perpetual conflict to provide the necessities of existence, utilize it as a means to diminish their burden and as a source of child or infant food. Any printed notice that such milk is unfit for such a purpose is a totally inadequate protection. Its consistency and concentration deceives the eye and masks its utter deficiency in fat, while the apparently fattening properties of the sugar bolsters up the initial deception. I do not know of any class who need such a variety of condensed milk, I am unaware of any section of the community who would be prejudiced by its elimination. In my opinion its manufacture in this country and its importation into it should be prohibited. This could of course be done by imposing a minimum fat standard.

While canned meats are much more uniform in composition the published analyses show a good deal of difference as regards their chemical composition. The two factors of importance which show the widest differ-

[1] In May 1923 the Ministry of Health issued Regulations (Circular 393) dealing with the labelling and composition of condensed milks, to come into operation on October 1, 1923.

ences are the fat which may vary from about 7 to 22 per cent. and the meat bases from o·62 to 1·47 per cent. according to U.S.A. Department of Agriculture figures. There seems no case at present for laying down standards as to composition, and indeed the subject requires more study, but the possibility must be kept in mind.

Considerable differences occur in regard to the relative quantity of fruit and syrup in canned fruits but at present the reputation of the canner or wholesale vendor seems to be sufficient protection.

WASTAGE OF CANNED FOODS AND UTILIZATION OF REJECTED TINS

The problem of the reduction of wastage from spoilage will be dealt with in Lecture II after the bacteriology of canned foods has been considered. It is only proposed to consider here its magnitude and the methods of disposal of rejected tins.

The total amount of canned food lost by the contents becoming unsound can be grouped under two broad headings, i.e. factory loss and post-factory rejections. I have tried on a number of occasions to obtain information as to the percentage loss at different factories but this is information jealously guarded and always denied to me. For one thing it varies considerably with season and from other causes. Some factories, even well equipped and well conducted ones will have a run of what is called "bad luck," which can really be more accurately described as undetected bad management and lack of attention to minute but essential details, and will turn out batches of canned foods a material percentage of which is spoiled. Speaking very generally canners tell me that they would only regard about o·5 per cent. of wastage as normal and anything beyond that unwarranted and demanding strict investigation.

The practice at the cannery as regards preliminary

incubation (i.e. storage in a warm room) of the tins before release materially increases the proportion of spoilage tins which can be grouped as factory spoilage and proportionately diminishes those which occur after the tins leave the cannery.

Post-factory wastage is the sum of the loss from rejections at the ports and other places of primary inspection and of spoilage in course of transit or storage detected by inspector, trader or consumer.

No comprehensive figures are available as to what this loss amounts to but some idea of its extent can be gleaned from the following figures dealing with canned foods condemned at certain places of entry and which I owe to the kindness of the Medical Officers of Health concerned.

TABLE IX

Food condemned (in cwts.).

Place	Year 1919				Year 1920			
	Meat	Marine	Fruit	Milk	Meat	Marine	Fruit	Milk
Port of London ...	630	101	397	842	1766	22	701	9790
Bermondsey ...	2442	166	1447	4139	6616	49	2556	5805
Southwark ...	2920	5	422	1438	498	95	995	4784
Stepney	1225	100	38	833	3301	76	1681	2646
Southampton ...	26	0	1	102	76	6	11	240
Manchester Port...	33	1	117	189	488	0	180	39
Bristol Port ...	153	0	33	133	391	1	10	219
Liverpool Port ...	461	19	178	363	200	10	408	77

Place	Year 1921			
	Meat	Marine	Fruit	Milk
Port of London ...	283	271	4764	530
Bermondsey ...	3061	52	5423	4121
Southwark ...	3063	60	668	4665
Stepney	3106	319	1532	1928
Southampton ...	24	84	21	23
Manchester Port ...	26	0	48	41
Bristol Port ...	157	0	248	356
Liverpool Port ...	189	5	137	7

In addition very large quantities are rejected in the areas of the different Sanitary Authorities after they have passed through the ports and wharves and been admitted, so to speak, into circulation. No complete figures are available but in the City of Liverpool (apart from the Port) in 1920, 23,314 and in 1921, 21,427 tins of canned foods were condemned as unfit for human consumption. In the City of London in 1921 the rejections were 535 cwt. tinned meat, 275 cwt. tinned milk and 231 cwt. tinned marine products. These two examples will give some idea how extensive the rejections are, after the tins have left the wharves.

The figures in the table show that for the four areas in London mentioned the loss from canned meat alone in 1920 was 12,181 cwt. or 1,364,272 lbs. If this is valued at a shilling a pound it represents an annual loss of over £68,000 from canned meat in these areas alone.

As regards the disposal and utilization of this vast quantity of condemned canned foods no uniform or comprehensive plan is adopted but each Local Authority makes its own arrangements for their disposal. The methods of disposal vary to some extent with the nature of the food to be got rid of. From inquiries made at the chief ports and places where large quantities of these foods are condemned it would appear that while a good deal of the meat is destroyed or dumped into the sea, a large part is released under definite restrictions for animal food, for manure and for fat extraction, about £3—4 per ton being obtained for it. Milk is largely utilized for pig feeding and to a lesser extent for poultry feeding but considerable quantities are destroyed. Fruit always and fish and other marine products commonly are destroyed or discharged with other refuse into the sea but a small proportion of marine products are used for pig feeding or for manure.

All the Medical Officers of Health concerned are fully alive to the importance of taking steps to ensure that this food should not be picked over and the least damaged or the apparently sound tins re-enter the markets by illicit means. When the tins are to be destroyed, and occasionally when they are consigned outside the area, one procedure is to pierce the tins before they leave the supervision of the condemning Local Authority. This however is only the practice in some areas. Often a guarantee is furnished by the user that none will be used for human food.

When the tins go into the area of another authority it is the usual practice to notify the Medical Officer of Health of the district of this fact, but it does not appear to be the usual custom to follow up the different consignments to ensure their use for the purposes alleged. Mere notification to the outside Local Authority Medical Officer hardly seems adequate to exclude the possibility of these tins being sorted over and some being utilized for food. In many cases they go into rural areas in which the Medical Officer of Health is in General Practice and not a Public Health expert, and who may not regard his duties more seriously than in proportion to the paltry salary paid him and who does not follow up the matter at all. It must be remembered that many of these tins are not obtrusively bad and are quite saleable.

It would certainly seem desirable that the business of the disposal of these vast numbers of rejected tins should be placed on a better basis. It is undesirable that each Local Authority be left to make its own arrangements. If there was common action a uniform procedure could be devised and acted upon and more satisfactory arrangements made for safeguarding against the possibility of condemned food being used for human food. The food which now has to be destroyed in the destructor or dumped into the sea could be used for animal food or other legitimate purposes and not wasted at heavy expense.

With tinned foods the main difficulty of utilization

is the cost of opening the tins and it is common sense that in such a centre as London there should be concentration of means of disposal, while supervision would be greatly facilitated. In the City of London where so much food is admitted and distributed the City Corporation has let a tender for several years for dealing with unsound food to one firm which has established the necessary plant. While the main supplies dealt with are raw foods large quantities of tinned goods are disposed of and Dr Howarth (*M.O.H.* 1921 *Annual Report, City of London*) in an interesting account states that the plant includes an electrically driven saw capable of opening 700 tins per hour. The company does not find it profitable to deal with tins of fruit or even condensed milk.

LECTURE II

THE BACTERIOLOGY OF CANNED FOODS

THE prevailing view, both scientific and popular, in regard to canned foods is that they are types of preserved foods which remain sound because the food is rendered sterile by the application of heat and maintained in that condition by being kept in hermetically sealed containers. The only exception recognized is as regards sweetened condensed milk which is admitted to contain some organisms, the keeping qualities being explained by the fact that a preservative (sugar) is added in large amounts which prevents these bacteria from doing any harm. When canned foods become unsound the explanation offered is either that the sterilization was inadequate or that the continuity of the tin was defective, admitting bacteria from outside which decomposed the food.

Two quotations from standard text-books may be mentioned showing that the above statement of current views is correct.

Marshall's *Microbiology*, 2nd Edition, 1917, referring to the spoilation of canned food states "microbial changes occur when the goods have not been processed at a temperature sufficiently high to destroy all the organisms which may have been present in the uncooked food."

Leach and Winton, *Food Inspection and Analysis*, 4th Edition, 1920, states "The preservation of food by canning was long thought to be due to the perfect exclusion of air, but is now known to depend on the perfect sterilization of bacteria, and it has been proved that as far as keeping qualities are concerned, it makes no difference whether or not air is present in the can, if the contents are sterile."

It will be shown conclusively that this simple conception does not represent the facts and that the factors which determine whether or not canned foods remain in a sound and safe condition are far more complex.

The first point of interest is an answer to the question, To what extent are sound canned foods sterile ? The following table gives the results of the detailed examination of a number of perfectly sound samples of various canned foods purchased in the open market in this country and which have been examined by my colleagues and myself during the last four years.

TABLE X

Sound shop samples

Product	No. examined	Sterile	Not sterile	Percentage not sterile	Percentage not sterile
Meat	22	8	14	63·6	
Salmon	16	8	8	50·0	
Sardines	11	7	4	36·4	Fish 48·6
Herrings	8	3	5	62·5	Marine products 61·1
Crab	10	0	10	100·0	
Lobster	6	1	5	83·3	Crustacea 84·2
Crayfish	3	2	1	33·3	
Fruit	58	45	13	22·4	
Unsweetened condensed milk[1] ...	44	36	8	18·2	
Sweetened condensed milk ...	15	0	15	100·0	
Excluding sweetened milk	178	110	68	38·2	

This table shows that while no class of product was always sterile the percentage varied from 18·2 per cent. not sterile for unsweetened milk to 84·2 for crustacea and 100 for sweetened milk.

Vaillard as long ago as 1900 found organisms in 70 to 80 per cent. of his samples, but his work was gener-

[1] Includes 17 "Factory" samples, i.e. sound tins just as they leave the cannery.

ally discredited and ascribed to faulty technique and outside contamination. Recently Weinzirl (1919) and Cheyney (1919) examined sound samples and found a percentage not sterile. Cheyney found the percentage not sterile to be corned beef 18, salmon 20, sardines 9, lobster 4, shrimp 8, crab 25, tuna fish 8, fruit 2·8.

My percentage of not sterile samples is considerably higher than either Weinzirl's or Cheyney's. Considerations will be advanced shortly which lead me to believe that even my high positive results are an understatement for at least some of these foods, particularly the marine products group, and that if more specialized methods were employed almost all the latter group would show the presence of living bacilli.

While to these investigators must be given the credit of first clearly demonstrating that many sound samples may contain living bacteria our studies have carried the matter much further and we have been able to demonstrate why these bacteria may be present without risk of spoilage. The significant feature is not the mere fact of the presence or absence of living bacilli but the types of bacteria which are present.

Are we to assume that these bacteria are all of types which are unable to decompose the food, and if any decomposition types are present then the food will invariably become unsound? In other words can we shift the standpoint and conclude that whether foods become unsound or not does not depend upon sterility but is conditioned by the presence or absence of bacilli of decomposing type.

This particular point was not dealt with by Cheyney and he confines his attention to pointing out that "the organisms isolated constitute a sharply limited group of resistant spore bearers." Weinzirl goes further and concludes that "the living spores found in commercial canned foods are unable to grow in the food, due to the absence of oxygen."

The following table (Table XI) summarizes the organisms which we have isolated from sound tins, omitting the sweetened condensed milk samples.

TABLE XI

Product	Yeasts	Obligate anaerobes	Sporing aerobes	Thermo-phils	Micro-cocci	Non-sporing bacilli
Meat	o	o	7	6	5	1
Salmon	o	o	3	3	4	1
Sardines	o	o	4	1	1	o
Herrings	o	o	3	3	o	o
Crab	o	2	2	9	3	o
Lobster	o	o	3	2	o	o
Crayfish	o	o	1	o	o	o
Fruit	1	7	10	o	o	o
Unsweetened milk	1	o	5	1	4	o
Total	2	9	38	25	17	2

Many of these organisms, as will be shown later, are capable of decomposing the food from which they were isolated. It is clear therefore that the problem of decomposition is not the simple one of the presence or absence of bacilli of decomposing type but the far more complicated one of ascertaining the conditions which will allow bacilli of this type to become active agents of decomposition.

The chief types of organisms isolated by us from a large series of rejected samples are shown in Table XII. They are grouped into two classes according as the contents were found to be unsound or apparently in good condition.

To be able to cause canned foods to become unsound microorganisms must possess certain attributes in addition to the ability to grow in these foods. One or other of the following must be a characteristic of their vital activity: proteolytic or fermentative properties. An organism with proteolytic properties is able under favourable conditions to decompose proteins with the production of secondary degradation products. If such

TABLE XII

Condition of contents	Types of organisms isolated	Food product									
		Meat	Salmon	Sardines	Herrings	Lobster	Crab	Crayfish	Fruit	Sweetened milk	Unsweetened milk
Unsound (including all with gas escape)	No. of tins examined ...	32	27	16	5	9	13	8	67	33	47
	Anaerobes	9	2	3	0	2	3	1	3	1	4
	Sporing aerobes (excluding thermophils) ...	11	9	4	2	2	4	3	9	33	7
	Thermophils	4	1	4	0	1	1	0	3	{10 (out of 16)	0
	Non-sporing bacilli of decomposing type ...	5	11	4	0	3	3	1	2	5	6
	Non-sporing bacilli of non-decomposing type ...	6	3	4	0	0	5	0	0	—[1]	2
	Coccoidal-bacillus type ...	0	0	0	0	0	0	0	16	—[1]	5
	Micrococci	13	10	3	4	3	7	1	14	33	21
	Yeasts	0	0	0	0	0	0	0	12	30	2
	Sterile	2	3	5	1	1	0	3	24	0	9
Rejected, but contents apparently sound	No. of tins examined ...	64	35	15	14	5	5	4	40	13	10
	Anaerobes	0	2	0	3	0	0	0	3	1	1
	Sporing aerobes (excluding thermophils) ...	8	6	3	4	1	0	1	5	12	1
	Thermophils	5	2	3	1	0	2	1	4	{9 (out of 10)	0
	Non-sporing bacilli of decomposing type ...	1	4	1	0	1	0	0	0	0	0
	Non-sporing bacilli of non-decomposing type ...	1	1	0	2	0	0	2	0	—[1]	0
	Coccoidal-bacillus type ...	—	0	0	0	0	0	0	1	—[1]	0
	Micrococci	7	6	2	3	2	1	1	5	13	0
	Yeasts	0	0	0	0	0	0	0	2	3	0
	Sterile	48	22	10	6	2	2	0	25	0	8

products include some which are gaseous the tin is likely to contain gas while the contents will be decomposed. The ability to produce gas from carbohydrates

[1] Not looked for in every sample.

or from bodies such as inosite is the other important characteristic. The property of producing acid, but without gas formation, from carbohydrates is of importance as regards condensed milks but otherwise is not of significance. If any particular organism possesses proteolytic or fermentative properties, still more so if it exhibits both functions, it must be classed as a potential cause of decomposition of canned foods. The converse is probably equally true; if any strain or group of organisms exhibits neither of these properties then we must regard it as unable to initiate unsoundness in canned foods other than milk. There is a possible exception to this statement. It is conceivable, and we possess some but rather inconclusive evidence that it may occur under actual conditions, that two strains neither of which by itself belongs to either group may by their symbiotic activities produce decomposition changes. From our results I consider this to be, at the most, a rare possibility.

In my canned food studies proteolytic ability was judged by the ability to liquefy blood serum under optimum conditions. Neither the production of indol, the formation of sulphuretted hydrogen nor the capacity to liquefy gelatine are reliable tests of proteolytic ability.

It is well known that the ability to decompose carbohydrate with gas production is materially influenced by the variety of carbohydrate, some organisms for example readily decomposing glucose but are unable to break down more complicated sugars such as saccharose or lactose. While many varieties of carbohydrates were tested by us, for present purposes I include any strain which can produce gas from glucose or other simple carbohydrate as possessing fermentative abilities.

To readily grasp the significance of the different types isolated it is of value to tabulate them from this point of view.

Type of organism		Proteolytic	Fermentative
Obligate anaerobes		+	+
Ordinary sporing aerobic bacilli ...		+(most strains)	−
Thermophilic bacilli		−(„ „)	−
Non-sporing aerobic bacilli	B. proteus group	+	+
	B. cloacae „	−	+
	B. coli „	−	+
	Glucose, non-lactose group	−	+
	Non-fermenting groups ...	−	−
Micrococci		−	−
Yeasts		−	±

From this grouping we should anticipate that the obligate anaerobes and the *B. proteus* types would give the most obtrusive signs of unsoundness, causing both a blown condition of the tin and offensive decomposition of the contents. The non-proteolytic but fermenting types of non-sporing aerobic bacilli would be prolific causes of a blown condition but the contents would not show much change, while similar results would be obtained with fermenting yeasts. The sporing aerobes should give rise to decomposition changes but not to a blown condition of the tin. The micrococci and most of the thermophils would be unlikely to cause either external changes in the tin or unsoundness in the contents.

Such a general conception of the activities of these different types of organisms does correspond fairly closely with actual findings but there are a good many exceptions and other factors have to be taken into consideration. The tables already quoted as to the distribution of the different types in sound and unsound tins show the extent to which exceptions are met with. For example sporing aerobic bacilli were as prevalent in sound as in unsound tins while anaerobes were occasionally found in tins with perfectly good contents.

That the proteolytic and decomposing types of bacilli

are capable of inducing decomposition changes in canned foods was amply proved by a long series of experiments in which perfectly sound tins were inoculated with such organisms in pure culture under aseptic conditions and the tins at once sealed up again. Two such inoculations may be quoted as examples.

Exp. A sound tin of salmon was inoculated with strain A 474, an anaerobic bacillus of Rauschbrand type isolated from an unsound tin. The tin was sealed up and incubated at 37° C. Gas developed within the tin and when opened after 43 days the contents were decomposed and had a putrid odour. The inoculated strain was recovered in pure culture.

Exp. A sound tin of beef was inoculated with strain A 268, a typical *B. coli* organism isolated from an unsound tin of meat. The tin was sealed up and incubated at 37° C. for 30 days. The container itself was markedly blown but the contents showed no, or but very insignificant, signs of decomposition. The inoculated strain was recovered.

It will be of interest and of practical value if each group of organisms is reviewed briefly as regards its prevalence in canned foods and as to how far it can be considered a cause of spoilage.

Yeasts. While occasionally isolated from meat or marine products they are of little or no significance as a cause of unsoundness in these products but are of great importance in connection with tinned milk and tinned fruit.

They are of most importance in relation to sweetened condensed milk and the following table sets out our results as to their distribution in this food.

Table XIII

Type of tin	No. examined	No. containing yeasts	Percentage containing yeasts	Percentage containing fermenting yeasts
Rejected and blown ...	33	30	91	71
Sound shop	15	4	27	0
Sound fresh factory ...	23	14	61	43·5
Sound incubated factory	15	11	73	53·3

A "factory" tin is a sound tin obtained direct from the factory where canned, the date of canning being known, and usually put up only a week or so before examination. Some were incubated in the laboratory for considerable periods and constitute the "incubated factory" group.

The type of yeast was carefully studied but the only characteristic of importance in these studies was whether or not it fermented glucose and saccharose. The nonfermenting strains were found to be of no significance as regards the development of spoilage. The table shows that fermenting yeasts were isolated from nearly all the blown tins, were absent from the shop tins but were present in nearly half of the freshly put up factory tins.

The ability of the fermenting types to cause gaseous decomposition in sweetened condensed milk was fully demonstrated in numerous experiments. It was equally evident that the mere presence of fermenting yeasts did not invariably cause gas to develop and the milk to become unsound, indeed their occurrence in sound tins was frequent. A long and elaborate series of experiments which are set out elsewhere[1] were necessary before we could elucidate the conditions necessary for decomposition to result. We demonstrated by special experiments that yeasts do not readily multiply in condensed milk tins, partly due to the medium being unsuitable but chiefly because of the restricted supply of oxygen. Before they can cause fermentation changes yeasts have first to multiply and for this they must be supplied with oxygen and the supply when the tin is closed is restricted. If only a few fermenting yeasts gain access they are unlikely to produce gas and cause the tin to become blown because they will not increase sufficiently before anaerobic conditions become established in the tin and in consequence their multiplication

---

[1] Studies in Sweetened and Unsweetened (Evaporated) Condensed Milk. 1923 Food Investigation Board. *Special Report*, No. 13.

activities be shut down. The two primary factors controlling their decomposition activities are either the initial presence of a considerable number of cells or conditions which give air access and so enable them to increase sufficiently and take on the fermenting rôle, when they are then comparatively independent of any oxygen supply.

In my experience yeasts are an unimportant cause of decomposition in unsweetened milk as they were only isolated from two out of 60 rejected tins, in but one of which were they the cause of the gas development or other unsound conditions found. In fruit tins they are of greater significance and fermenting yeasts were found as a cause of unsoundness in 13 out of 107 cases.

Micrococci. Micrococci of various kinds, streptococci, staphylococci, diplococci and occasionally sarcinae, mainly owe any interest they possess in relation to canned foods to the fact that they are frequently present. Their percentage prevalence in our series of examinations is shown in the following table.

TABLE XIV

Canned food	No. of tins examined	Percentage prevalence in			
		Sound tins	Rejected tins with good contents	Unfit samples	All samples
Meat	116	23	11	40	21
True fish	142	14	17	39	22
Crustacea	64	15	33	37	30
Sweetened condensed milk...	95	100	100	100	100
Unsweetened condensed milk	104	9	0	45	24
Fruit	165	0	11	24	12

These organisms, devoid as they are of any proteolytic or fermentative properties under ordinary conditions, are of no significance as a cause of unsoundness as regards meat, "marine products" and sweetened condensed milk. In unsweetened milk we have been able to demonstrate the rather remarkable fact that under certain conditions some of our strains were able to produce gas. Most of them produce acid and I regard micrococci as an important cause of spoilage in this variety of food. In fruit we did not find them in sound samples but they were present in 24 per cent. of blown unfit tins. Although numerous experiments were carried out to elucidate the position the results obtained were somewhat inconclusive. They suggest as probable that at least some of the strains must be held responsible as causes of unsoundness in tinned fruit.

Anaerobic sporing bacilli. We have abundant evidence that these organisms are important causes of spoilage of canned foods. The tables however show that these bacilli were sometimes isolated from perfectly sound tins. Anaerobes were isolated from two perfectly sound shop crab tins, from a sound salmon tin (not included in the table) and from five rejected tins with quite good contents (two salmon, three herring). Since they were all strongly proteolytic and decomposing types and the anaerobic requirements are satisfied by the conditions which exist in the tins this is a fact which is unexpected and difficult to explain. I was only able to explain it after a great deal of special experimental work. Cheyney only found an anaerobe once (crab) in 725 cans of merchantable food and Weinzirl not at all in sound tins.

Even more striking results were obtained in a further series of experiments. Seventeen perfectly sound tins of different marine products were given air access through punctures (but only sterile air was admitted through cotton wool plugs) and incubated in that condition for 5–16 days and then sealed up again and re-incubated. The results obtained after the final opening are summarized in the following table:

TABLE XV

	Marine product	No. examined	Contents		Sporing aerobes	An-aerobes	Other organisms
			Good	Unfit			
Punctured	Lobster ...	3	1	2	3	1	0
	Salmon ...	6	0	6	5	2	3
	Crab ...	1	1	0	1	1	0
	Sardines ...	2	2	0	2	0	2
	Herrings ...	5	1	4	5	5	4
	Total punctured	17	5	12	16	9	9
Not punctured	Salmon ...	2	2	0	0	0	0
	Herrings ...	2	2	0	0	0	0

With the exception of two cases the contents of the nine tins containing anaerobes were unfit. All the anaerobes were proteolytic and fermentative. In this series no less than 53 per cent. of the tins contained living anaerobes. These experiments suggest that a considerable proportion of these sound tins of marine products contain spores of anaerobes but in a dormant condition.

From the numerous experiments initiated to investigate the anomaly it appears probable that the survival of a few scanty spores of these anaerobes is not uncommon, at least in marine products. They are incapable of multiplication if only complex proteins are available. When the tins are given air access the sporing aerobes also present grow and their proteolytic enzymes elaborate simpler protein degradation products which enable the dormant anaerobic spores present in turn to multiply. The deeper parts of the contents are still anaerobic and, once they have started, their own enzymes can continue the dissolution of the proteins.

Sporing aerobic bacilli. Owing to their wide distribution in nature, their high resistance to heat and the almost inevitable contamination of canned food products with members of the group the significance of the presence of these organisms in canned foods is of great practical moment. Their importance has been mostly overlooked until our studies.

Table XVI shows how frequently they were found. This table shows their *percentage* prevalence in tins with sound and unsound contents.

TABLE XVI

Contents	Anaerobes		Sporing aerobes		Fermenting non-sporing aerobes	
	Sound	Unsound	Sound	Unsound	Sound	Unsound
Meat	0	28	32	30	0	16
Marine	4	14	30	31	0	28
Fruit	12	4	14	13	0	3
Unsweetened milk	0	9	11	6	0	13
Sweetened milk ...	0	3	87	100	7	15

The table shows that they were just as prevalent in sound shop samples as in tins with definitely unfit contents. Not all the members of the group are proteolytic but the great majority are, although many only liquefy blood serum slowly. Out of 91 strains isolated from meat and marine products all but 14 were proteolytic and the strains which liquefied blood serum were just as prevalent in the sound shop tins as in tins with unfit contents. It is usually stated that these organisms will not grow under anaerobic conditions but we were able to isolate many strains which grew well under ordinary anaerobic conditions and even fairly well under the strictest anaerobic conditions I could devise. While they could grow, a series of experiments showed that they did not do so with sufficient facility to produce enzymes capable of peptonizing milk or liquefying blood serum.

Table XV shows that sporing aerobes were isolated from 16 out of the 17 punctured tins. In eight cases they were the only decomposing proteolytic strains isolated and five of these eight tins showed unfit contents. In a long series of special inoculations we were able to show that inoculating a sound tin of meat or fish invariably caused decomposition of the food when air access was permitted but that this result only occasionally followed after inoculation when the tin was immediately sealed up.

It is evident that these organisms are very widespread in some canned foods and, at least as regards meat and marine products, in a far higher proportion than our results from simple examinations show. They are present as spores and remain dormant and unimportant under the ordinary anaerobic conditions provided in properly sealed cans. Supplied with air the spores develop into vegetative forms and produce enzymes which decompose the food. In other words the proteolytic members of this group are potential causes of decomposition of canned foods.

Non-sporing bacilli of decomposing or fermenting types. Their percentage distribution is shown in Table XVI. They include many types and are important causes of decomposition changes.

The *B. proteus* group possess both fermentative and proteolytic properties and in consequence cause the retainers to become blown while the contents are decomposed. They were isolated almost entirely from meat and marine products.

Organisms of the *B. cloacae* type caused considerable gas development but only slowly developed changes in the food. They were most frequently isolated from lobsters but were also found in unsweetened milk.

B. coli was only rarely isolated from meat tins but was comparatively common in blown tins of marine products, particularly salmon. Here no doubt it gained access from contaminated water.

This surmise has been shown to be the case, as regards decomposing salmon, by Hunter (1922). He studied the bacterial groups in decomposing salmon and concluded that the bacteria concerned have their natural habitat in the sea-water from which the salmon are taken and that the decomposition is not due to bacteria which contaminate the salmon within the cannery.

B. coli was also found to be a cause of decomposition in unsweetened condensed milk but although it was isolated seven times from sweetened condensed milk it was unimportant as a cause of decomposition. It was found twice in fruit as a cause of gas development. Being devoid of proteolytic properties its effects are most noticeable as gas production, the food itself showing very little change.

In fruit a peculiar and special type of bacillus was found as an important cause of unsoundness. This was a remarkably pleomorphic organism which in ordinary culture media grew as a coccoid bacillus, only slightly longer than broad, but which in fruit juice grew out into a long slender bacillus. It grew well under both aerobic and anaerobic conditions. All the strains isolated were devoid of proteolytic properties and under ordinary conditions none decomposed any carbohydrate. A special series of experiments demonstrated that this organism does produce gas when introduced into sound tins of fruit and that such tins become "blown." All the strains produce a large amount of acid but the gas development is not due to the action of this acid upon the tin but to direct fermentation of the fruit juice. I have not found this organism described elsewhere or previously recognized as a cause of fruit decomposition and have called it *B. pleofructi*. As many as eighteen strains were isolated, in every case from a tin which was defective and usually with the contents unfit. I consider this unusual type of bacillus to be a common cause of unsoundness in fruit.

We have also isolated the same organism from five unsound tins of unsweetened condensed milk and have been able to demonstrate its ability to decompose that fluid. The organism is non-pathogenic to mice and guinea-pigs.

Thermophilic bacteria. These are all sporing aerobic bacilli the characteristic features of which are their ability to grow at temperatures considerably above those favoured by ordinary bacteria and that their optimum growth takes place at these high temperatures. Some are obligate thermophils and are unable to multiply at 37° C. or lower, but others are facultative and while they grow best at 55° C. or thereabouts they can multiply at 37° C.

We have found them to be widely present in canned foods as shown in the following table from our own results.

TABLE XVII

Canned food	No. of tins examined	Percentage prevalence in			
		Shop and factory	Rejected but good contents	Unfit contents	All samples
Meat	41	27	54	25	34
Salmon	54	21	8	0	9
Sardines	36	9	28	14	25
Herrings	27	37	7	0	15
Crustacea (crab, lobster, crayfish)	58	58	20	13	28
Sweetened milk	47	62	90	81	77
Unsweetened milk ...	100	2	0	0	1
Fruit	165	0	9	5	4

None of them possessed any fermentative properties and only a few any proteolytic ability. Direct inoculation experiments failed to cause decomposition and they seem to be of little or no significance as a cause of spoilage.

It will be seen that the facts which have been ad-

vanced from four years' close study of the bacteriology
of these foods suggest conclusions at variance with the
usual views. It will be evident that they have a very
practical bearing upon the whole subject of the spoilage
of canned foods. It may be helpful to briefly summarize
these views and explain their influence upon the practice
of canning.

SUMMARY OF BACTERIOLOGY OF CANNED FOODS IN RELATION TO SPOILAGE

It would appear that a large proportion of canned
foods as put upon the market, and which are sound and
wholesome, are not sterile. The proportion not sterile
varies from 100 per cent. for sweetened condensed milk
to 18–20 per cent. for unsweetened milk and fruit, according to our findings. There are reasons to believe
that the figures given are an understatement. Further,
many of these organisms differ in no way from strains
which we have shown can and do cause marked spoilage,
under other conditions, in the same kinds of food products. In other words the conditions under which they
are found are at least of equal if not of greater importance than their mere presence. Of such conditions the
two which are of greatest significance are the conditions
within the tin as regards the availability of free oxygen
and the initial number of the organisms present.

All our results emphasize the essential importance
of absolutely airtight retainers, not because outside
bacteria may get in but because the admission of air
may provide conditions suitable for the multiplication
of bacteria *already present*. Even obligate anaerobes
(paradoxical as it sounds) may be stimulated to become
actively decomposing organisms by the introduction of
air. The number of living organisms is also a factor of
material moment. It is difficult for a few spores to start
and multiply and produce sufficient enzymes to furnish
the simpler protein products requisite for abundant

growth. Given enough of them this process is facilitated and nothing more may be required. It is evident that the prevention of spoilage is not a simple but a highly complicated matter.

The practical conditions to ensure a minimum of spoilage are in my opinion the following:

(*a*) As small initial bacterial contamination as possible.

(*b*) Conditions within the factory which allow as little bacterial multiplication as possible before the tins are hermetically sealed up.

(*c*) A processing[1] temperature which will at least ensure only the survival of spores and as few of these as possible.

(*d*) A satisfactory form of container and reliable methods of closure which will ensure and maintain a perfectly airtight tin.

It might be supposed that with the demonstration of the frequent absence of sterility in canned foods it should be a simple matter for the food canner to alter his methods and arrange that the temperature to which he submits his finished product is one which will ensure the destruction of all bacteria whether in the vegetative or sporing form. Only a superficial study of the technical and trade side of this vast business is necessary to realize that such a simple solution is impracticable.

The technical problems involved in processing are complex and are discussed at some length in Appendix I. This Report shows that it is not simply a question of the application of so much heat to "process" the product but this factor is influenced by a number of physical laws making it a complicated and technical subject.

The facts explained in Appendix I show how im-

[1] The expression "processing" is the technical term applied in the trade to the final heating given to the product in the can after it has been sealed up. It is better than the word "sterilization," which is sometimes employed as its equivalent, as the latter implies the definite view that all bacteria have been destroyed, an implication which is not in accordance with the facts.

practicable it is to set out precise data in regard to time and temperature of processing which are generally applicable. It is only within the last few years that any serious attempt has been made to remove the subject from one of empiricism to one on a scientific basis and much yet remains to be done.

The prevention of spoilage depends upon many factors, including the reduction of the number of bacteria introduced by only using clean fresh material quickly handled under scrupulously clean factory conditions, an accurate adjustment of the degree of heat and its time of operation to the particular foodstuff, and the use of thoroughly sound containers sealed in an efficient manner with complete exclusion of air.

As regards spoilage one cannot help feeling that the canner has been fortunate. He has aimed at sterility and, because most of his products remained sound, fondly thought he had attained it. He relied on his processing to produce sterility and upon an airtight tin to keep out germs from what he believed was a sterile product. But he builded better than he knew. He has by no means attained sterility but fortunately has reached something which is nearly as good. Provided his workings are rapid and clean and he uses fresh stuff he has attained to the condition of leaving only a few living organisms, mostly as spores, in a food product not very nutritive when not broken down, stored in an airtight receptacle. Under such conditions the living bacilli mostly remain dormant. If he cannot ensure this dormant condition spoilage results in many cases.

CHANGES WHICH OCCUR IN SOUND FOOD AFTER CANNING.

The extent to which changes take place in food after canning, when the food is and remains perfectly good, is a subject of considerable importance to the trade but one in regard to which very little is known scientifically. It might be supposed that if the food is sterilized and air is excluded that no changes would occur, apart from any action upon the metal retainers. Direct examination, however, shows that considerable changes may result, but that their degree and nature vary with the product. In canned meat little or no alterations take place or at least none appear to have been reported. With fruit changes are comparatively slight, apart from solution of tin and iron through the action of the acid juice upon the retainer. The most definite changes occur with milk and marine products.

The changes in condensed milk occur in both the sweetened and unsweetened varieties but are more definite in the former kind. We have paid considerable attention to their nature. Sweetened condensed milk is never sterile and one change is an alteration in the numbers and kinds of bacteria present. In an unopened airtight tin the general tendency is for a gradual decrease to take place in the total number. Some organisms appear to slowly multiply but this is offset by a decrease in the viability of others until a rough equilibrium is established.

If however the tins are not airtight the results are in marked contrast. In a long series of experiments the result was a very great increase in the total number of organisms, which reached its maximum after about two to three weeks at 21° C. or after a considerably shorter period at 37° C. and then a steady decline, so that at the end of three or four months the number of organisms present was less than at the start. Some variation occurred but nearly all followed this general plan. The feature of great bacterial increase with air access may be of significance in connection with infant feeding as opened tins of sweetened condensed milk are frequently used for infant feeding for many days and until the contents are all used up.

Two striking changes with time which are markedly accelerated as the temperature rises, are a progressive thickening and darkening of the milk, the two changes being concurrent but not proportionate to one another. These changes may be so marked that in old tins, especially if kept in tropical climates, the milk may be nearly solid and of the colour of chocolate.

The thickening is undoubtedly due to colloidal changes in the concentrated milk. It has been suggested that they are due to bacterial enzymes but my investigations do not support this view. The increase is in no degree proportional to the bacterial content. The studies of Rogers, Deysher and Evans (1920) led them to conclude that the casein is the constituent principally concerned in the production of the increased viscosity and that one of the factors greatly increasing the tendency to thicken is the temperature used to heat the milk preliminary to its condensation. Viale and Rabbeno (1921) have recently studied the chemical changes and report considerable alterations including a gradual hydrolysis of the proteins, hydrolysis of lactose and sucrose to monosaccharides and saponification of neutral fats. These changes only become considerable after several years of storage.

In canned marine products, especially herrings and sardines, definite changes occur on storage. Such canned fish mature and do not attain their best condition for some time, which may be several years. As Professor Johnstone (1921) puts it, "The crude and 'raw' taste characteristic of the freshly packed fish disappears on maturation. The bones become soft and very friable (though the scales never do become softer than in the newly packed fish). The flesh becomes soft and pasty, so that the fish easily breaks when taken from the tin. The smell changes. The flavour of the fish improves very notably, of course, and this is the result which is desired from maturation."

Johnstone discusses the cause of maturation. In an earlier report (1919) he suggests that these alterations, which have nothing in common with putrefactive changes, are not bacterial but are an autolytic process due to specific intracellular enzymes not entirely destroyed by sterilization. In his later report (1921) he points out that the possibility of bacterial action cannot be negatived while he also considers the possibility that the process of maturation is the consequence of a catalytic action in which organized enzymes are not involved. On this supposition the tin taken up would act as a catalyst.

Weber and Wilson (1919) have shown that packs of sardines upon standing show a marked increase in the quantity of total volatile nitrogen, the greater part of which is in the form of amines.

They found that storage caused a gradual increase in the volatile bases and in the organic acids and this was greater the higher the temperature of incubation, being very small indeed at $0°$ C. The presence of *purée* greatly increased the rapidity of formation of the volatile bases but the organic acids increased to a greater extent in the specimens containing no *purée*. The variations in the amount of amino-acids during the six months' period of observation were less regular and decreases occurred in the first four weeks, the content rising subsequently.

Storage at a temperature of $33°$ F. greatly retarded their formation. The relative quantities of ammonia and amines composing the total volatile alkaline material changed during storage. After processing practically two-thirds of the total alkaline nitrogen consisted of ammonia and one-third of amines. After storage these proportions changed to about equal parts of each. Storage at a low temperature while causing a decrease in the total quantity of ammonia and amines apparently does not affect the relative amounts. Most of the volatile alkaline material existed in the form of trimethylamine in stored canned sardines. They also investigated the development and causation of blackening or detinning of the inner surface of stored unlacquered sardine tins. They found it more developed with skinned than with unskinned sardines. They ascertained it was due to sulphide of iron and concluded that the ammonia and amines in solution are the main cause.

Foreman and Miss Marrack (1922) working with canned herrings have studied this question in connection with other problems. Their work is at present incomplete but is suggestive that these maturation changes are due to the activities of bacteria which have survived the processing given.

The subject needs much more investigation but in view of our results as to the survival of bacteria in these fish after processing it seems probable that these changes are in the main due to the action of enzymes produced by the activities of bacteria which have resisted the sterilization after canning.

While it is theoretically possible that changes with storage in tins with sound contents and which remain good may result in the formation of products which are directly inimical to man on ingestion, there is no evidence that any such products are ever produced. These changes are worthy of extended investigation from the point of view of the value and palatability of the food product but are of very minor significance in relation to problems of injury to health.

LECTURE III

DIRECT RELATIONSHIP TO DISEASE
CONDITIONS

I PROPOSE in this lecture to consider in some detail to what extent there is any direct evidence that the consumption of canned foods is a cause of disease or malnutrition amongst the community. In Lecture I it has been pointed out that the consumption of these foods has increased enormously and is likely to increase still further. It is to be anticipated that a change of this magnitude in the habits of the community should have some influence upon the public health. Popular prejudice exists to a considerable degree against canned foods and there is an inclination amongst the unscientific to accept the most trivial and inadequate evidence as pointing unmistakably to special danger from their consumption. In the lay press this attitude is only too common and when sudden illness of a gastro-intestinal type occurs, should canned foods have been eaten any time shortly before the development of symptoms, the immediate bias is to lay the blame upon such food. Coroners' Courts are thickly strewn with verdicts casting unsubstantiated imputations upon canned foods.

It is of great importance therefore to consider critically, impartially, and with care the ways in which such food may be prejudicial and exactly the evidence that is available showing that prejudicial effects have resulted. It is perhaps necessary to point out that there are really two considerations involved. One is the extent to which any danger to health is merely common to the type of food used and is independent of this special method of preparation. The other the existence of any detrimental effect which is peculiar to canned foods and definitely associated with this class of product. Both considerations have to be borne in mind in discussing the problem.

Scientifically considered any possible menace to health may be classified into the following groups:

1. *Bacterial.* As carriers of living pathogenic bacilli or their toxins. From incipient putrefaction or other general bacterial unsoundness.

2. *Parasitic.* As carriers of living animal parasites.

3. *Chemical.* From the presence of inorganic chemical poisons, either added in the course of manufacture or derived from the retainers.

4. *Loss of accessory food factors.* From the loss or diminution of vitamins or other food factors necessary to the human organism.

It will make for clarity if these groups are discussed separately.

Bacterial infection or toxin poisoning. The different bacterial conditions which may give rise to infection or illness through the vehicle of canned foods fall conveniently into three classes.

Group A. From bacilli specifically associated with outbreaks of food poisoning.

Group B. From other pathogenic bacilli.

Group C. From bacterial infection, or toxaemia, from decomposed or putrefactive food.

The specific food poisoning bacilli fall into two groups as a matter of convenience, i.e. Salmonella group organisms and *B. botulinus.* The resultant outbreaks are so different in character that they are best dealt with separately.

FOOD POISONING OUTBREAKS DUE TO CANNED FOODS, APART FROM BOTULISM

The problem of botulism is separately considered. Apart from that condition there is no doubt that food poisoning outbreaks may originate from the consumption of canned foods but there is a good deal of difference of opinion as to the extent to which they occur. As already mentioned, the popular view in this country is one of considerable suspicion towards this type of food. For some years I have been on the look out for food poisoning outbreaks of all sorts and particularly those associated with canned foods and have tabulated in Table XVIII 51 such outbreaks. It is important to explain that only outbreaks in which there is a strong probability, and in most a definite certainty, that the vehicle of infection was the canned food are so included. Almost all the cases in recent years have been personally inquired into and many of them I have bacteriologically investigated. I think all those in the Table can be definitely included as due to the consumption of canned foods. A considerable number of so-called canned food outbreaks has been excluded from consideration as either decidedly negative or so indefinite as not to warrant inclusion. Particulars of one such outbreak definitely ascribed to canned foods without warrant may be of interest. On a Saturday a family of five had mid-day dinner which included a one pound tin of corned beef the contents of which excited no adverse comment. One of the family, a child of four, was ill next day, seriously ill on the Tuesday, a doctor was called in on the Thursday, and the child died on the Friday. The father was said to have suffered from abdominal pains and the mother from slight diarrhoea, both on the Sunday, but were well next day. The other two children ate the same meat but were not ill in any way. A post-mortem on the child disclosed acute peritonitis and no intestinal disease. No bacteriological examinations were made. The symptoms of the fatal case were not those of food poisoning and there was no vomiting until the Wednesday night. Although this was confidently put down to food poisoning from canned food there is no evidence of any food poisoning. The child died of acute peritonitis and the indefinite and slight symptoms of the parents were probably as much suggested by the illness of the child as by anything else.

That 51 definite outbreaks in this country can be collected shows that this vehicle of food poisoning cannot be neglected, while during the four years (1919–1922) when I was specially on the watch for them 29 outbreaks were collected. It must also be taken into consideration that the food poisoning outbreaks which attract attention are those in which a death occurs and publicity is given by an inquest. The majority of outbreaks from canned foods are due to toxins and very rarely cause a fatality. Quite certainly many such outbreaks are overlooked and never come to official notice, since there is no obligation to report them to Health Officers.

In relation to the actual amount of canned foods consumed the number of poisonous tins is extremely small and probably less than 0·0001 or even 0·00001 per cent. but their actual total number is far from negligible and much greater than it should be.

To discuss the subject in detail would be to traverse the whole problem of food poisoning and it is only possible here to draw attention to a few points which specially concern this vehicle of infection.

In almost all cases the canned food consumed, although toxic, has been indistinguishable in appearance, odour or taste from sound canned food. The illness is not due to the consumption of decomposed or abnormal food. There is no evidence of poisoning from ptomaines or any products of decomposition. It follows that in nearly all cases there is no means of safeguarding the consumer either by more detailed and rigid examination of canned foods on importation or by a more careful discrimination by the consumer as to only eating sound tins with seemingly sound contents. The safeguard offered against botulism is here absent.

In all these tabulated outbreaks there is no evidence of chemical poisoning from tin, etc., although such a contingency may occur in rare cases.

In these canned food outbreaks, in certainly the vast majority of cases, the cause of the illness is the same as when the vehicle is some other type of food, i.e. to infection with a member of the Salmonella group of bacteria. The illness is due either to infection with a living bacillus or to undestroyed toxins. When due to canned foods the characteristic feature is the high proportion due to toxins only, no living bacilli being present. This is what might be anticipated since the "processing" given is usually adequate to kill non-sporing bacilli like the members of the Salmonella group but may be insufficient to destroy their toxins which are known to possess marked resistance to heat.

The evidence is not adequate to affirm that all the outbreaks in Table XVIII are due to Salmonella bacilli or their toxins but the greater number can with confidence be so ascribed. I have endeavoured to group the outbreaks from this point of view into three classes, i.e.:

(*a*) Due to living bacilli, probably or certainly of Salmonella group = 16 outbreaks.

(*b*) Due to undestroyed Salmonella group toxins = 27 outbreaks.

(*c*) Information inadequate to ascribe accurately to (*a*) or (*b*) = 8.

In class (*a*) a Salmonella bacillus was only isolated eight times but in the other half adequate bacteriological examinations were not carried out. From the long incubation period, the fact that a death often resulted and other details it is possible to conclude with certainty that a living bacterium was the cause of the outbreak.

The 27 outbreaks in class (*b*) are grouped as due to toxins because in some cases it was possible to demonstrate positive agglutinins in the blood of the sufferers while in the others the short incubation period, characters of the symptoms and other features of the outbreak make this type of causation probable. There are considerable difficulties in the way of proving the etiological association when toxins are the cause. Some are technical in character and Mr Bruce White and I are carrying out experiments with a view to their elimination.

The influence of season is distinctly less noticeable in food poisoning outbreaks due to canned foods than when the vehicle is fresh food. Of 106 outbreaks of food poisoning including all vehicles which I have collected

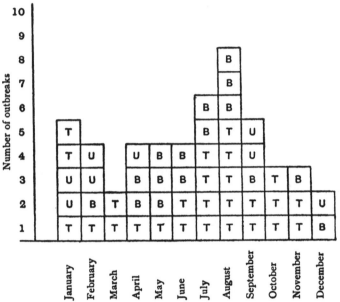

Chart 1. Seasonal distribution of 47 canned food poisoning outbreaks. Great Britain only.

T = due to toxins only.
B = due to living bacilli and toxins.
U = Information inadequate to decide.

49 per cent. were in June, July or August while in the 51 canned food outbreaks 18, or 35 per cent., were in those months. As the chart shows they exhibit only a moderate increase of prevalence in the warmer months.

This is what might be anticipated since the seasons of consumption need have no relationship to the season of distribution of infection with canned foods, although the activity of the toxins may be greater in warmer weather. It is probable that more canned foods are eaten in the summer which may increase the incidence then. For the 16 outbreaks in which living bacilli were present in the canned foods the percentage prevalence in the three summer months rises to 44.

The vehicles of infection were as follows :

```
Meat (Beef 20, Mutton 1, Tongue 5)...26
Salmon ...      ...      ...      ...   ...16
Other fish (Herrings 1, Sardines 1)  ... 2
Crustacea      ...      ...      ...   ... 2
Fruit    ...      ...      ...      ...   ... 5
```

A study of the individual outbreaks in which canned meat was the vehicle shows that four were due to living bacilli, 19 were due to toxins only, while in the others the information and investigations were inadequate for a decision. Meat is usually "processed" at temperatures high enough to kill the bacilli but not always high enough to destroy the heat-resisting toxins of the Salmonella group, so the high proportion of "toxin" outbreaks is readily understandable.

The place of packing is not available for all these canned meat outbreaks but of the 14 more recent ones (1919–1922) in 10 this is known and in every case the infected meat was packed in South America. It is true that much of our imported canned meat comes from this Continent but Table III (Lecture I) shows that only 53·5 per cent. so imported came from South America. This point is rather striking and definite, and suggests either that undetected or unexcluded Salmonella infections are more common in South America or else that the temperature-time period of processing there is less satisfactory than in other places of manufacture.

The salmon outbreaks on the other hand were much more commonly due to infection with living bacilli. Although living Salmonella strains were actually only isolated from two, in 8 of the 16 outbreaks deaths resulted and this and the other facts showed infection with living bacilli. In only six outbreaks can the cause be ascribed with confidence to toxins and all of these were during the last two years. In earlier years these less severe outbreaks were probably overlooked or at least not reported in the press. The lower "processing" temperatures employed for salmon will account for this difference between the proportion of living bacilli to toxin outbreaks exhibited by salmon and meat vehicles.

While I have particulars of a few outbreaks in which several tins of one particular consignment have been infected this is the exception. One of the most striking examples of this was in connection with an outbreak in 1910 at St Helens and elsewhere due to toxins only. The consignment was a very large one comprising thousands of tins. One six pound tin at St Helens was sold in August in small lots to eleven families and 32 out of the 33 who ate it were attacked. Other individual tins caused 21 cases at Carlisle in the same month, 6 at Gateshead in September and 15 at Hessle in November. In each instance one tin only in each place seemed to be affected. There were no deaths, although many of the sufferers were very ill.

My experience is that it is usual for only a few tins (indeed in most cases only one) of a consignment which may run into 10,000 or more tins to be infective. In numerous instances I have examined numbers of such tins without finding any more of them to contain harmful bacilli or toxins. In all these outbreaks, with the rarest exceptions, the facts are conclusive that the food was not infected after opening and we can be certain that the bacilli or their toxins are survivals from infection already present at the place of canning.

TABLE XVIII

Food poisoning outbreaks from canned foods

Serial no.	Place	Year	Month	Incubation period (in hours)	Number of cases	Deaths	Tinned food eaten	Animal from which food derived	Living bacillus isolated	If evidence of Salmonella toxins alone
1	Oldham	1882	—	½—5	9	0	Tongue	Pig	No	—
2	Wolverhampton	1884	May	10—14	3	2	Salmon	Salmon	—	—
3	Sheffield	1899	November	1—3½	24	1	Beef	Ox	*B. enteritidis*	+
4	Partick	1906	May	1—4	12	0	Salmon	"	No	—
5	Tunstall	1907	April	10—14	3	1	Salmon	Salmon	—	—
6	Longton	"	August	12—24	4	1	"	"	*B. enteritidis*	—
7	Banff	1909	June	2—6	16	0	Beef	Ox	—	—
8	St Helens	1910	August	2—10	32	0	"	"	—	—
9	Astley	"	"	1	7	0	Tongue	?	—	—
10	Burslem	"	"	7—8	4	1	Salmon	Salmon	—	—
11	Newcastle	"	December	—	19	1	Mutton	Sheep	*B. aertrycke* (Newport)	—
12	Newcastle, Battle Hill	"	"		5	0	Salmon	Salmon	—	—
13	Chester	1911	March	½—6	10	0	Beef	Ox	—	+*B. enteritidis*
14	Walthamstow	"	September		7+	1	Tongue	?	—	—
15	Wigan	"	"	2	11	0	Beef	Ox	—	—
16	Skelmanthorpe	1914	February		5	1	Peaches	—	Gaertner	—
17	Liverpool	1915	January		18	0	Salmon	Salmon	—	—
18	Bradford	1918	February	½—5	3	1	Salmon	Salmon	—	—
19	Tamworth	"	"	5—48	10	0	Beef	Ox	—	—
20	Bordon	"	April		102	0	Salmon	Salmon	—	—
21	Bradford	"	January		1	0	Herrings	Herring	Gaertner	—
22	Southampton	1919	"	1—2	9	0	Beef	Ox	—	+*B. aertrycke* (m.)
23	Dunfermline	"	February	—	3	0	"	"	No	—

No.	Place	Year	Date	Interval	Cases	Deaths	Food	Food	Bacteriology	Result
24	London	1919	May	a few hours	1	1	Sardines	Sardines	No	—
25	Tipton	"	July	6	4	1	Salmon	Salmon	No	—
26	Birmingham	"	"	2	4	0	Crayfish	Crayfish	"	—
27	Glasgow	"	August	2½—4	18	0	Tongue	Ox	"	Indefinite
28	Bristol	1920	"	18—48	63	1	Beef	Salmon	*B. aertrycke* (Newport)	
29	Newcastle-on-Tyne	"	July	—	?		Salmon	Salmon	—	—
30	Glasgow	"	August	2—3	7	0	Beef	"	—	
31	Barrow-in-Furness	"	September	12 (average)	42	2	Salmon	Ox	*B. aertrycke*	—
32	Glasgow (Kelvin)	"	November	1½—2½	24	0	Salmon	"	—	Inconclusive
33	Nottingham	1921	March	½—5 (2—3 most)	9	0	Salmon	Salmon	—	Neg.
34	Birmingham	"	May	about 24	4	1	Tomatoes	—	*B. aer-trycke* (m.)	—
35	Falkirk	"	July	1½	3	0	Salmon	Salmon	—	—
36	Penarth	"	August	4	18	0	Tongue	—	Neg.	+*B. aertrycke*
37	Preston	"	October	3	5	0	Salmon	Salmon	"	Neg.
38	Aberdeen	"	November	1—2	30	0	Beef	Ox		+*B. aer-trycke* (m.)
39	Stafford	"	January	4	2	0	Tomatoes	—	"	—
40	Trowbridge	1922	April	under 2	2	1	Prawns	Prawns	"	+*B. aer-trycke* (m.)
41	South Shields	"	June	15—19	4	1	Salmon	Salmon	"	Neg.
42	Larbert	"	"	1½	5	0	Beef	Ox	*B. aer-trycke* (m.)	—
43	Bristol	"	"	long	4	1	Apricots	—	Neg.	
44	Liverpool	"	July	2½—3½	16+	0	Beef	Ox	"	Neg.
45	Chester	"	"	1—1½	4	0	Salmon	Salmon	"	+
46	Middlesborough	"	September	2—4	22	0	Beef	Ox	"	Neg.
47	Rosewell	"	"	7	3	1	Pears	—	"	"
48	Chesterfield	"	October	2	6	0	Salmon	Salmon	"	"
49	Newcastle-on-Tyne	"	"	about 2	over 32	0	Beef	Ox	"	"
50	Kettering	1923	January	2½—3½	about 12	0	"	"	"	"
51	Birmingham	"	"			0	"	"	Indefinite	Indefinite

My own conception of what occurs is that, under conditions which we have insufficient knowledge to define with precision, some of the meat, salmon, etc., becomes infected with living Salmonella group organisms. It is a well ascertained fact that oxen, pigs and other animals used for canned meat suffer from infection with members of this group and this is probably the source of the bacilli in these cases. For salmon, however, I know of no such infection but that may be because it has not been investigated. The infection of the meat or fish is limited, and results in only a small proportion of tins of any one batch becoming specifically infected. The sterilization processes given are probably adequate to destroy the bacilli in all but a tin or two which are insufficiently heated, due to faulty packing in the retorts, etc. The same applies to the toxins, but as these possess considerable heat resistance they are more likely to survive.

Such infective tins do not become unsound externally, nor do the contents decompose, and their existence cannot be detected other than by a bacteriological examination of the actual tin. It is fortunate that the number of infected and poisonous tins is not more numerous than it is since they are undetectable by any precautions which can be adopted by Food Inspection Authorities. The only way to prevent the occurrence of such outbreaks is by the elimination of these bacilli at their source. One would like to know to what extent Salmonella group infections occur amongst cattle used for canning in South America and whether this group of bacilli can be found in salmon used at the great salmon canneries. This is all part of the larger subject of food poisoning generally and cannot be discussed in greater detail here.

BOTULISM

First reported in Germany and in adjacent parts of Europe this variety of food poisoning was usually associated with the consumption of sausages, ham, smoked fish and the like, and it is only in the last decade that outbreaks of this character have been associated with the eating of canned foods. Since 1907 there has been a considerable number of these outbreaks from canned foods, and almost invariably in California and other parts of Western U.S.A. The first bacteriologically demonstrated outbreak in America was in 1914, the vehicle being cheese. Meyer and Geiger, writing in 1921, mention since 1900, 39 human outbreaks in California, with a probable total of 130 cases and a mortality of 94 cases (72·3 per cent.). This disease is not confined to man, but one type of *B. botulinus* (Type A of Burke) affects fowls, and the other type (Type B) causes disease in horses (so called "forage poisoning"), and during the same period there have been reported 42 outbreaks in fowls and 79 in horses, making in all 160 outbreaks in California. A certain number of outbreaks is likely to be overlooked, or at least not reported, and the figures suggest that in California there now exists an endemic focus of this disease. Table XIX gives particulars of 84 outbreaks in U.S.A. or Canada all from canned or bottled foods. They comprise 319 cases with 206 deaths, a case mortality of 64·6. Of these outbreaks 52 were home, 31 commercially canned and 1 was doubtful.

In a paper read at the Plymouth Congress in June 1922 and published in July I wrote:

"In view of the enormous quantities of tinned fruit canned in that State which reach this country it is worthy of consideration as to how far there is a possibility of the introduction of botulism into this country."

TABLE XIX

Outbreaks of Botulism from canned and bottled foods.—U.S.A. and Canada

No.	Year	Place	Number of		Tinned or bottled food vehicle	Home or commercial canned	If bacteriologically proved
			Cases	Deaths			
1	1906	Los Angeles, California	3	3	Pork and beans	Com.	—
2	1910	Oroville, California	4	4	String beans	Com.	—
3	1910	Sawtelle, California	11	11	Pears	Home	—
4	1910	Yakima Valley, Washington State	6	3	Asparagus	Home	—
5	1912	Amador City, California	6	5	String beans	Home	—
6	1912	San Jose, California	2	1	Clam juice	Com. (bott.)	—
7	1912	Romley, Colorado	7	5	Spinach or String beans	Com.	—
8	1913	Palo Alto, California	12	1	String beans	Home	—
9	1913	San Francisco, California	3	2	Clam juice	Com. (bott.)	Yes
10	1914	Spokane, Washington State	2	2	Clam juice	Com.	—
11	1915	Fallbrook, California	5	5	Apricots	Home	—
12	1915	Sacramento, California	1	1	Asparagus	Home	—
13	1915	Hillsboro, Oregon	1	1	Corn	Home	Yes
14	1915	Basalt, Colorado	5	5	String beans	Home	—
15	1915	Chicago	2	2	Pimientos	Com.	Yes
16	1915	Salt Lake, Utah	1	1	Asparagus	Home	Yes
17	1916	San Jose, California	1	1	String beans	Home	Yes
18	1916	San Pasquale, California	1	0	String beans	Home	—
19	1916	Yakima Valley, Washington State	1	1	Corn	Home	—
20	1917	Escondito, California	7	4	String beans	Home	Yes
21	1917	Corning, California	1	0	Corn	Home	Yes
22	1917	Seattle, Washington State	3	3	Asparagus	Home	Yes
23	1917	Yakima Valley, Washington State	1	1	Corn	Home	—
24	1917	Ontario, Oregon	1	1	String beans	Home	—
25	1917	New York State	7	5	Corn	Home	—
26	1918	Madera, California	8	6	Apricots	Home	Yes

No.	Year	Location			Food	Source	
27	1918	Los Angeles, California	1	1	String beans	Home	—
28	1918	Oakdale, California	1	1	String beans	Home	—
29	1918	Fresno, California	1	1	String beans	Home	Yes
30	1918	Napa, California	2	2	(Minced) Olives	Com.	—
31	1918	San Bernardino, California	2	0	Apricots	Home	—
32	1918	Colton, California	1	0	Pears	Home	—
33	1918	San Rafael, California	1	1	Corn	Com.	—
34	1918	Los Angeles, California	1	0	Tuna	Com.	—
35	1918	Yakima Valley, Washington State	4	4	Corn	Home	Yes
36	1918	Boise, Idaho	7	4	Asparagus	Home	Yes
37	1918	Decatur, Indiana	1	1	String beans	Home	—
38	1918	Klamath Falls, Oregon	3	2	String beans	Home	—
39	1918	Newark, New Jersey State	4	4	String beans	Home	—
40	1918	San Rafael, California	1	1	String beans	Home	—
41	1919	Los Angeles, California	1	1	String beans	Home	—
42	1919	McKenna, Washington State	3	3	Spinach	Home	Yes
43	1919	Canton, Ohio	14	7	Olives	Com. (bott.)	Yes
44	1919	Detroit, Michigan	7	5	Olives	Com. (bott.)	Yes
45	1919	Yava, Montana	7	5	Olives	Com. (bott.)	—
46	1919	Dawson City, Canada	23	12	Beets (?)	Com.	—
47	?	Chicago	2	0	Tomato catsup	Com. (bott.)	Yes?
48	1920	Oakland, California	6	3	Spinach	Com.	Yes
49	1920	Richmond, California	1	1	Olives	Com.	Yes
50	1920	Los Angeles, California	1	1	String beans	Home	—
51	1920	Los Angeles, California	1	0	String beans	Home	—
52	1920	Los Angeles, California	5	0	Olives	Com.	—
53	1920	Los Angeles, California	4	1	(Minced) Olives	?	—
54	1920	Yakima Valley, Washington State	1	1	Milk	Com.	—
55	1920	Walla Walla, Washington State	5	5	Asparagus	Home	Yes
56	1920	New York City	7	7	Olives	Com. (bott.)	Yes
57	1920	Memphis, Tennessee	3	3	Olives	Com. (bott.)	Yes
58	1920	Greensbury, Pennsylvania	3	5	Olives	Com. (bott.)	Yes
59	1920	Florence, Arizona	5	5	Beets	Com.	Yes

Table XIX (*continued*)

Outbreaks of Botulism from canned and bottled foods.—U.S.A. and Canada

No.	Year	Place	Number of Cases	Number of Deaths	Tinned or bottled food vehicle	Home or commercial canned	If bacteriologically proved
60	1920	Pittsburgh, Pennsylvania ...	4	3	Corn	Home	—
61	1920	New York City ...	2	2	Spinach	Com.	—
62	1921	San Diego, California ...	1	0	Spinach	Com.	Yes
63	1921	Seattle, Washington State ...	1	1	String beans	Home	Yes
64	1921	Yakima Valley, Washington State	1	1	Corn	Home	Yes
65	1921	Yakima Valley, Washington State	2	2	Spinach	Home	—
66	1921	Yakima Valley, Washington State	1	1	Corn	Home	Yes
67	1921	Grand Rapids, Michigan ...	29	3	Spinach	Com.	Yes
68	1921	Battle Creek, Michigan ...	5	2	Spinach	Com.	Yes
69	1921	Mischawaka, Indiana ...	2	2	Spinach	Com.	Yes
70	1921	Pueblo, Colorado ...	5	3	Beets	Home	—
71	1921	Parkersburg, Virginia ...	1	1	Pumpkin	Com.	Yes
72	1921	Grants' Pass, Oregon ...	1	1	String beans	Home	Yes
73	1922	San Tacinto, California ...	1	1	Fish (pickled and bottled)	Home	Yes
74	1922	Canaan, Ohio ...	2	2	Spinach	Com.	—
75	1922	San Francisco, California ...	2	2	String beans	Home	—
76	1922	Cambridge, Idaho ...	8	6	Turnip tops as "greens"	Home	—
77	1922	Healdsberg, California ...	3	3	String beans	Home	Yes
78	1922	Weiser, Idaho ...	1	1	String beans	Home	Yes
79	1922	Kendallville, Indiana ...	9	4	Corn	Com.	Yes
80	1922	Cheyenne, Wyoming ...	1	1	Corn|	Home	—
81	1922	Toppenish, Washington State ...	1	1	Corn	Home	Yes
82	1922	Templeton, California ...	1	0	String beans	Home	—
83	1922	Starbrick, Washington State ...	4	4	Asparagus	Home	—
84	1922	Watsonville, California ...	2	2	Chili sauce in bottles	Home	Yes

Within a month of its appearance the dramatic and very fatal outbreak at Loch Maree occurred. The following is a brief account of this outbreak.

On August 14th, 1922, amongst some 48 persons staying at Loch Maree Hotel in the Highlands of Scotland six guests and two ghillies ate for their lunch sandwiches made from a certain jar of potted meat paste. Two meat paste pots were used to make the sandwiches that morning but only one was poisonous, a jar of wild-duck paste. Nothing unusual as to its condition was noticed by the cook who made the sandwiches. All but one of the cases were attacked the next day, the remaining person becoming ill on the morning following. They lived for different periods but all eight died with the characteristic symptoms of botulism. *B. botulinus* (Type A) was isolated by Mr Bruce White from the traces of paste left, and from remains of one sandwich, while the presence of the characteristic toxin was demonstrated in both remains. The facts exclude infection at the time of opening and the toxins must have been forming there for some time. Although the methods of manufacture and conditions of cleanliness at the factory were very good one can only postulate that some stray infection must have taken place there during manufacture, or before manufacture, and have escaped sterilization. Only this one solitary jar out of the whole batch appears to have been infected or at least to have remained infective after sterilization.

The literature of botulism is now so considerable, largely due to the industry of American workers, that to review it would occupy more than one lecture. In Table XIX is set out a tabular statement of outbreaks in which the vehicle was preserved (canned or bottled) food. This table is compiled from information furnished me by Dr Meyer and I am greatly indebted to him for permission to use this material and before he has utilized it for publication. I propose here to indicate the salient facts, so far as they relate to canned foods, so that conclusions can be drawn as to the extent of the danger and the precautions necessary to remove risk of botulism being induced from the consumption of such foods.

The primary seat of *B. botulinus*, the organism responsible for these outbreaks, is the soil. Dr K. F. Meyer[1] and other investigators have been able to show that spores of this organism are not only widely distributed in U.S.A. but are also present in old world soil and they have isolated it from Belgium, Denmark, the Netherlands, Switzerland and England. Out of 64 soil samples from England which in 1921 I transmitted to California to Dr Meyer for examination five showed the presence of *B. botulinus* (8 per cent.) and two others showed weakly toxic cultures (11 per cent. in all). In certain parts of America it is more widely distributed in the soil and in California Meyer and Dubovsky[1] found it in 45 out of 78 samples of virgin soil (57·6 per cent.) and in 59 out of 226 samples of garden, orchard and cultivated field soil (26·1 per cent.). They make the highly important observation that the bacillus is found in greatest abundance in soil that has never been cultivated and that it is less prevalent in more cultivated regions. They add: "It is evident that in California at least *B. botulinus* is not disseminated by animal excreta nor is the intestinal canal the natural habitat of this organism."

The spores of this bacillus have also been isolated from fruits and vegetables bought in the open market in California, and Meyer and Dubovsky[1] out of 122 such samples found 33 (27·0 per cent.) produced toxic cultures.

In view of these facts and its isolation from spoiled

[1] Information from as yet unpublished papers kindly placed at my disposal by Dr Meyer of California.

canned foods in California and other countries the possibility of outbreaks from these foods imported into this country cannot be ignored. The canned goods which have most commonly served as the vehicle are vegetables and to a lesser extent fruits, but meat pastes and other made up meat foods may also so act.

An estimate of the danger of this disease being caused by canned foods can only be given after the following considerations have been discussed. These will be dealt with *seriatim.*

1. Is the bacillus so widespread that material contamination of the foods used in canning is likely? The facts enumerated show that in areas where the soil is heavily contaminated a percentage of fruit and vegetables can be shown to harbour this organism. Nearly all these bacilli would be washed off in the preliminary processes but some might remain and, for example with tomatoes, I have seen them not only initially heavily contaminated with soil but visible soil has been left on them when they have passed through the washing stages and been put into tins. I have no doubt that a very important factor is the use of quite fresh and unbruised fruit or vegetables. *B. botulinus* thrives in decaying food and in incipiently decomposed food there is an added likelihood of multiplication of this organism and a lessened liability to dislodgment in the subsequent cleansing stages.

2. Is the "processing" given adequate to ensure the destruction of *B. botulinus*, whether in the spore or bacillus form, and of its toxin? The bacillus readily succumbs to heat and its toxin is comparatively thermolabile; the temperature of boiling water will easily and rapidly destroy both. It is safe to assume that the ordinary processing given, if adequately performed, will destroy these. The spores are however vastly more resistant. The earlier accounts, including the work of Van Ermengen, suggest a low resistance and

30 minutes at 80 °C. were found to destroy them, but the later American work shows a high degree of resistance. Weiss (1921), for example, finds that their thermal death point in canned foods varies with the hydrogen ion concentration of the particular food. The more acid foods, such as canned fruits, require a maximum of 50 minutes at 100° C. or 15 minutes at 110° C. while with the less acid vegetable products up to 180 minutes at 100° C. or 10 to 20 minutes at 110° C. may be required. The most recent investigation is that of Esty (1923). He studied 112 strains, 37 of which were derived from human outbreaks of botulism. The heat resistance of these strains varied from 3 to 75 minutes at 105° C. when heated in a phosphate solution of approximately P_H 7·0. The heat resistance of the Type A strains varied from 3 to 75 minutes and those of Type B from 3 to 60 minutes. The average heat resistance of all strains was 41·1 and 23·8 minutes for Types A and B respectively, indicating that the majority of these spores are destroyed within a comparatively short time. Certain spores were very resistant. In general, young spores, particularly of the first generation, were the most vigorous and difficult to destroy. The heat resistance is also dependent upon the concentration of the spores. Enormous variability of the same strains to produce resistant spores was noted. The maximum heat resistance of *B. botulinus* spores, produced under optimum conditions of growth, in this phosphate medium was 330 minutes at 100° C., 110 minutes at 105° C., 33 minutes at 110° C., 11 minutes at 115° C. and 4 minutes at 120° C. He found spores of *B. botulinus* more resistant than those of any of the other anaerobes tested.

Their resistance is affected by other factors in the food besides acidity including their consistency and the concentration of the syrup. The age of the spores is also of considerable importance.

These facts are of great practical significance since

they show a degree of resistance which would enable at least some of the spores to survive the processing temperatures which are generally employed for these classes of foods. It is not impossible to employ degrees of heat which will ensure the destruction of these spores without damage to the quality of the food but it is certainly very difficult, and at present is not attained. The whole question is now being intensively studied but at present we must adopt the standpoint that if spores of *B. botulinus* are present in the unheated product the heating likely to be given to the sealed tin cannot be relied upon as invariably adequate to destroy these spores.

3. If the spores of *B. botulinus* survive in a preserved food, will the consumption of that food set up botulism? From the data supplied in Lecture II it is evident that two possibilities may occur, i.e. the spores may remain as such or may develop into bacilli and produce toxins.

Whether the spores remain dormant as spores or not depends on factors such as the number added, the temperature of incubation, the size of the tins and the hydrogen ion concentration. If they do not multiply the contents are usually non-toxic. Spores free from toxin can be fed to animals without harm, but if they are very numerous experiments show they may set up botulism. This probably only occurs if they are sufficiently numerous to contain enough intracellular toxin to poison the animal, or the positive results may be due to insufficient freedom from the toxins. There is no evidence that I can find that the spores under such conditions can germinate in the animal intestine or elsewhere and develop toxins.

In my own experiments with canned fruits the introduction of *B. botulinus* spores, unaccompanied by bacillary forms, caused no changes in the tins or the contents; they did not multiply and the contents were not toxic, if care was taken to introduce the spores free from toxin. On the other hand, in a certain proportion of cases the spores do develop into bacilli and if that occurs the food will be highly poisonous. In a food such as the wild-duck paste of the Loch Maree outbreak any introduced spores which remained alive are far more likely to multiply than in such a product as canned fruit, since in the former the conditions are so much more to their liking.

4. If the food contains *B. botulinus* toxin, will the tin show physical deviations from the normal, and will the contents be obtrusively altered? This question follows naturally from the two contingencies first mentioned. It is evident that undeveloped spores will originate no physical changes in the tin or contents but then poisonous toxins will be absent and the contents harmless.

B. botulinus is a proteolytic organism and a gas producer so that theoretically the development of the spores should invariably be associated with both physical alterations of the container (a blown or springy condition) and with decomposition changes of the contents. While in nearly all cases these theoretical results do accrue this is not invariably true and in a few outbreaks, notably from tinned spinach, no record of any sign of spoilage was made by anyone connected with the opening of the tin, preparing it for use or consuming it. This particular point needs further investigation particularly as to how far toxin production is antecedent to the development of the products of decomposition. It is evident that the likelihood of obtrusive changes being overlooked is greater for highly spiced or flavoured articles such as wild-duck paste than for simpler articles such as fruits or vegetables.

We have also to distinguish between slight changes only perhaps evident to the expert and definite physical alterations patent to even the most casual and ill-informed. A study of very many of the recorded outbreaks suggests to me as probable that deterioration changes are invariably present in a tin or jar with toxic contents but that while these are clearly demonstrable by the expert, they may sometimes be missed, although probably not often, by the ordinary cook or casual consumer. In this connection the Loch Maree outbreak is instructive. The inquiries just after the outbreak produced no evidence that the jar was unsealed or that the contents were obtrusively unsound. When, however, a sound tin of the same batch of paste was artificially inoculated with the Loch Maree strain in our laboratory, considerable gas developed which disturbed the paste and the smell was quite definitely altered. Although we have no direct evidence, since only such traces of paste were available for examination, that the peccant pot was physically altered I have no doubt definite changes had taken place and would have been noticeable to an expert.

From the answers to these four questions it is possible to draw some definite conclusions.

(a) The resistance of *B. botulinus* spores to heat is so considerable that it is very doubtful if absolute security is going to be attained by any system of sterilization. No manufacturer will so cook his food as to make it unmarketable and absolutely safe temperatures come somewhat near to it. It must also be remembered that "processing" is a procedure much governed by human considerations. Some batches are hurried through because they are urgently wanted or because the operative is in a hurry. Bad packing in the retorts may mean unequal heating and insufficient heating in some parts. Some fruits and vegetables are over-ripe or put into the tins in such a condition that in the operative's words "they will not stand much processing." Heating to a safety point may result in the spoilage of the lot and the process man is blamed: by somewhat underheating his risks in this direction are lessened or obviated. While much can be done to prescribe "safe" temperatures I am entirely sceptical of the possibility of yielding absolutely "safe" results as regards setting up botulism by any complete reliance on "processing" as a safeguard. The sterilization given must of course be absolutely sure to kill vegetable forms and toxins, but this is easily secured.

(*b*) Experience shows that after all *B. botulinus* is rare on foodstuffs. The selection of sound fruit and its use quite fresh with scrupulous cleanliness at all stages will very markedly reduce the risk. As already pointed out, decomposing food furnishes a nidus of growth for this anaerobe and the number of spores which have to be killed is a fundamental factor.

(*c*) In almost all cases the food which contains toxins of *B. botulinus* is obtrusively unsound. Anyone who deliberately or carelessly uses a spoilt tin of canned fruit or vegetables is disregarding a valuable warning and safeguard. With highly spiced foods this safeguard is more likely to be overlooked.

(*d*) A sense of proportion is necessary. In all Europe only about 74 outbreaks have been recorded while in the United States of America since 1899 up to the end of 1922 there have only been 110 outbreaks with 395 cases from all sources, while those from canned foods have been less than 90 outbreaks, that is in 22 years in a population of over one hundred million. In this country there has been one outbreak and only one. For 18 years I have been studying food poisoning, including this type, and carefully searching the literature, and the Loch Maree outbreak is the only recorded one I have been able to trace. Since that outbreak some newspapers would have us believe it is not so uncommon but the headlines do not correspond with the facts. Several of these so-called cases have been investigated under my supervision and all with negative results. The possibility of botulism from canned or other foods is a real one but the actual risk is infinitesimal.

INFECTION FROM OTHER SPECIFIC BACTERIA

Apart from the special food poisoning bacteria the risk of bacterial infection from canned foods is slight and the subject does not require any detailed consideration. The chance of the addition of such bacilli in process of manufacture is small and therefore the problem reduces itself to one of the extent to which the operations of canning reduce any risk inherent to the food in its fresh state. Canned foods are mostly cooked foods. Organisms like *B. typhosus*, *B. dysenteriae*, *B. diphtheriae* have a low heat resistance and the possibility of their presence and survival in canned foods is negligible and there are no recorded outbreaks, so far as I am aware, from infection of canned foods with these bacilli. Only two pathogenic organisms require separate mention and both in reference to condensed milk. While theoretically tuberculosis carcases might be used for meat canning the chances of any tubercle bacilli surviving the heating given are very small and canned meat can be considered free from living tubercle bacilli.

The evidence as to the survival of tubercle bacilli in condensed milk is inadequate for a definite statement. Delépine (1914) using tuberculous milk made into sweetened condensed milk found that the pasteurization given did not always kill the tubercle bacilli but the tuberculosis produced in guinea-pigs developed more slowly than in untreated milk. Other stages of the process would not affect the viability of any surviving tubercle bacilli. As I read his report his results show a material reduction in the number of surviving tubercle bacilli but not complete destruction, so that some may be left in the finished article. It is really all a matter of the time and temperature of the heating given to the milk before its condensation. If adequate no tubercle bacilli should survive and certainly the process generally can be accepted as markedly reducing the risk of

tubercle bacillus infection if it does not remove it altogether.

The other bacterial possibility is in connection with
streptococci. My experiments[1] show that under certain
conditions the streptococci always present in sweetened
condensed milk may increase markedly. It is possible
that some may be pathogenic and such condensed milk
be directly harmful for infant feeding. The risk, if any,
is probably less than with fresh milk.

This section can be summed up generally by saying
that the risk of infection from these pathogenic bacilli
is common to the foods when fresh but is very greatly
reduced and usually eliminated by the methods of preparation.

THE DANGER TO HEALTH FROM CANNED FOODS WHICH SHOW SIGNS OF DECOMPOSITION

The conception is so widespread, and so important
if it is true, that the use of unsound food, whether fresh
or in cans, for human food is fraught with serious
danger to health that it deserves and requires more
than passing attention. It has been shown that the
danger from canned foods containing the specific bacilli
of food poisoning or their undestroyed toxins is a real
and an important one. It has, however, also been
pointed out that, apart from the remote danger of
botulism, such food is almost invariably sound to the
physical senses and contained in receptacles which show
no deviation from the normal. The danger that is
apprehended here is something quite different and arises
either from the use of foods which are decomposed when
put into the tin or from foods which have become
unsound in the interval between canning and their
consumption.

The possibility is of peculiar importance for canned

[1] For details see Report on Studies in Sweetened and Unsweetened
Condensed Milk. 1923 Food Investigation Board, *Special Report*, No. 13.

foods for two reasons. In the first place there is a
liability that such food may be used. This particularly
applies to fish, which not only is a readily perishable
foodstuff but one which the nature of the methods of
collection make a possible contingency. A good deal
of the fish canned is collected by outside agents who
are paid according to the quantity and quality of the fish
delivered. It may have to be brought from considerable
distances and sufficient will have to be collected before
it is worth while to deliver it to the canneries or the
cannery boats. The fish first caught may begin to decompose but the whole catch is sold and, unless special
discrimination is shown, the whole catch is used. This
possibility is realized by the canners as a whole and the
modern tendency is to bring the canneries into closer
and closer proximity to the fish grounds.

The other point is that it is practicable to use unsound fish or other material for canning purposes and
yet on account of the heating given to supply a finished
product which will not decompose further in the tin
and which superficially will present the appearance
and other physical properties indistinguishable from
food made of the soundest material.

Before considering possible dangers to health it is
of interest to consider whether it is feasible to detect,
by any readily utilizable methods of examination, that
slightly decomposed products, particularly fish, have
been used in making the canned food. My experience
has shown me that many tins of fish or crustacea may
contain numerous living bacteria and be undesirable as
food but which, when opened, show surprising little
deviation from soundness as judged by the physical
senses. Some readily applicable chemical or other tests
would be of great value since bacterial cultivation
methods take many days and a decision within an hour
or so is what is wanted. Mr Hunwicke and I have
carried out a great deal of experimental work upon this

problem[1] and although we have obtained data of considerable comparative value our results do not by any means solve the difficulty. Mr F. W. Foreman and Miss Marrack are also working on this problem and by the use of improved methods are obtaining valuable information. It will not be possible to discuss these results in detail, but the whole of the data will be published separately. It is as yet extremely difficult to demonstrate the use of unsound food in canned articles if the subsequent sterilization given to the food has been adequate.

These various considerations make it of primary importance to investigate critically the possible dangers to health from the use of such food, both when subsequently sterilized and when it has not been sterilized but contains the living bacteria of putrefaction such as may be met with in tins which have become unsound after leaving the cannery. Stated in its simplest form it is a question as to the degree of toxicity of tainted or even definitely putrefactive food. The view which credits decomposed food with toxic properties largely rests upon a misconception due to the isolation of non-specific poisonous bodies called *ptomaines* from decomposing food and then assuming that these bodies which are toxic by injection, and not at all or to a very limited extent by feeding, are the cause of food poisoning. The isolation of split protein products of more definite composition, such as β-imidazolethylamine (histidine) and tyramine, in the intestine by the activity of putrefactive bacilli does not supply stronger information since although these bodies are highly toxic by injection under the skin, this evidence is not based on their toxicity by feeding, while they are found in the *normal* intestine.

I have attacked the problem (1921) on the direct practical side and have fed a series of kittens with extremely putrid mixtures of canned meat and fish over long periods and without demonstrating any definite

---

[1] Report not yet published.

signs of toxicity. I am unaware of, and have been quite unable to find, any evidence in favour of the popular conception as to the great toxicity of incipiently putrid food or even definitely decomposed food. I do not suggest it is harmless, but merely that there is no evidence available as to its harmfulness and its toxicity is in my opinion enormously exaggerated. There is no evidence of any scientific value that the general public runs any risk of illness from this source.

Such a view does not imply an acquiescence in the use of stale or unsound food for canning or that such use is free from risk. On the contrary I am strongly of opinion that a primary desideratum in canning is the use of foods which are cleanly collected, initially sound and used quite fresh. Such a belief is however not based on any hypothetical danger from the ingestion of the unspecific decomposition products contained in, or derived from, such stale or unsound food but is for two quite different reasons. One is that such food leads to spoilage and so the waste of valuable food, while the other is that such faulty conditions favour bacterial infection which may include the special bacteria associated with food infections and favour the multiplication of such specific bacteria. The risk of this has been pointed out in the section on botulism. The direct danger to health from canned food is not putrefactive and non-specific bacterial changes but the risk of infection with the specific bacteria associated with food poisoning.

ANIMAL PARASITES

The possibility of the conveyance of animal parasites through canned foods does not require detailed consideration. Any danger is confined to meat or almost entirely so confined. As regards meat the main parasites of importance are the tapeworms and trichina. A careful examination of the animals to be used for canned meat should detect the pathological condition and cause the rejection of the meat. Should however the meat be used, the heating to which it is subjected before placing it in the cans and the sterilization in the cans afterwards should be adequate to kill all living animal parasites. I am unaware of any cases of infection with animal parasites being traced to conveyance by canned foods. In other words, while meat used for canning like any other form of meat may be infected with animal parasites, the danger of canned meat acting as a vehicle for the living parasite is much less than with fresh meat because on the one hand supervision is likely to be more complete, and on the other because the cooking to which it is subjected is a reasonably reliable safeguard, although not an absolutely safe one.

CHEMICAL CONTAMINATION

Preservatives are not added to ordinary canned foods although they may be found in some meat essences and in some bottled foods. Their use is only incidental in canned foods and any discussion on them would be out of place. In the same way the use of copper salts in bottled peas or other vegetables is a very restricted problem and mostly confined to food packed in glass and need not be discussed. Dr Willoughby has recently drawn attention to the large quantities of copper sulphate in tinned spinach arriving at the Port of London, while still more recently copper sulphate has been found in *tinned* peas. More attention may have to be paid to these bodies in the future, but at the present time the only inorganic chemical substance which demands serious consideration is tin contamination and its possible danger to health.

The possibility of tin poisoning from the use of canned foods is one which has received considerable attention. Any risk of lead poisoning (from solder, etc.) is negligible and does not require separate discussion. The whole subject of the presence of tin in canned foods is discussed in detail in a valuable report by Buchanan and Schryver (1908) so that detailed consideration here is unnecessary.

There is no doubt that considerable quantities of tin may be removed from the retainers and incorporated in the food. Schryver summarizes the results of some 130 analyses of different canned foods, most of which had been kept a considerable time, in the following table:

Foodstuffs containing	Number	Percentage of total
Less than 1 grain per pound	72	55·4
Between 1 and 2 grains per pound ...	35	26·9
Between 2 and 3 grains per pound ...	17	13·0
More than 3 grains per pound ...	6	4·6

For further tabular information in regard to quantities of tin found in canned foods the very comprehensive report of the special American Technical Committee (1917) may be consulted.

The most important factors which govern the solution of the tin appear to be the nature of the food canned, the period since canning and the quality of the tin plate used.

Canned fruits, meat extracts and some marine foods are all products liable to contain considerable amounts of tin. With fruits and meat extracts the acidity of the liquid is an important factor but it is not the only one, and even with tins of the same age the amount of tin taken up is not proportional to the acidity. Investigations by Goss (1917) led him to conclude that large amounts of tin may be removed with foods of relatively slight acidity owing to the fact that the dissolved tin is constantly removed from solution by the proteins, carbohydrates and other substances present, the acid being regenerated and so capable of dissolving more tin. Goss, in common with Wirthle and other workers, found that in canned foods which consist of both solid and liquid portions the solid portions may come to contain relatively larger proportions of tin than the liquid. Using artificial tin digestion experiments, he found that the greater part of the tin was in an insoluble form and so firmly adsorbed that it will be eliminated directly from the body and not act physiologically as a soluble tin salt. Bigelow (1916) had previously come to the same conclusion. The longer the period since canning the higher the proportion of insoluble tin.

The presence of considerable quantities of tin in canned marine products is to some extent explained by the results of Bigelow and Bacon (1911). Examining canned shrimps they found monomethylamine in considerable amount and ascertained that this had a corrosive action on the retainers. They also concluded that the volatile alkalis and aminoacids in asparagus, spinach, string beans, etc., which strongly attack tin retainers have an effect analogous to the methylamine found in shrimps. Quite recently Foreman and Marrack (1922) have pointed out the considerable quantities of tin dissolved by tomato *purée* added to canned herrings. The *purée* is highly acid in character. One specimen of canned herrings seven years old was found to contain as much as 9·6 grains of tin per lb.

As regards direct evidence of toxic effects Schryver collected a few outbreaks in which poisoning resulted and which were ascribed to poisoning by tin. None are recent and the evidence that tin was the cause is not convincing in many of the cases. It is somewhat significant that few or no cases have been reported during the last decade or so. The consumption of tinned foods has enormously increased of recent years and if there exists any material danger of this metallic poisoning there should have been a corresponding increase of cases of poisoning from tin in canned foods.

Buchanan, in the report already quoted, suggests that when as much as two grains to the pound are found, the food should be regarded with grave suspicion and as potentially deleterious to health.

The available facts suggest that while the danger from tin poisoning cannot be ignored it is unimportant as a cause of illness unless very old tinned goods are sold. Quite recently, for example, in a food prosecution case at Southport as much as five and a half grains of tin per pound were found in a tin of tomatoes and the evidence was in favour of the view that the food had been packed for a considerable time. It was an instance of an acid fruit kept in a tin for a long time.

In view of the increase with age the possibility of tin poisoning is a sound argument in favour of the dating of canned goods and the rejection of old stocks of those foods which are known to have a considerable action upon tin plate.

It might be mentioned that with acid foods if the food is left in the tin after opening there may be an appreciable increase in the amount of tin taken up even after one day's storage, and this increases the longer left. With other foods tin solution is very slight or absent for several days.

VITAMINS AND CANNED FOODS

No consideration of the relationship of canned foods to health would be complete without some discussion as to the extent to which vitamins are injured or destroyed by the processes of canning.

Their existence in canned foods is not merely a question of whether they have been destroyed by heat, but also of their stability, for it is now recognized that they are not very stable bodies and are influenced by oxidation processes, while canned foods may be kept for long periods.

Also as regards these accessory substances quantitative considerations must be kept in mind, it is not merely a question of presence or absence. We not only require vitamins but must have a sufficiency of them, and if any preparation processes materially reduce the amount it may be nearly as prejudicial as if they were entirely destroyed.

It will be simplest to consider separately the information which is at present available in regard to the effects of heat on the different vitamins.

Fat soluble A accessory substance. The chief food containing it which is canned is milk, but a certain amount is contained in fresh meat, particularly internal organs such as liver and heart, in fish fat and in some vegetables and fruits.

The evidence as to the stability of the A vitamin is not altogether concordant but it would appear to be fairly heat stable. Osborne and Mendel (1915) found that butter fat treated with steam for two and a half hours did not lose its fat soluble A vitamin. Steenbock, Boutwell and Kent (1918) found that this vitamin is gradually destroyed at 100° C. In the special report by Halliburton, Paton, Drummond and others (1918–19) it is stated that experiments show that the fat soluble accessory factor is more thermolabile than was previously supposed to be the case. They tested whale oil heated to 100° C. and 150° C. for four hours respectively and in both cases the destruction of Fat soluble A was almost complete. Preliminary experiments with butter indicate that temperatures of 75–100° C. are sufficiently high, if continued for several hours, to cause destruction of Fat soluble A. On the other hand, still later work suggests that any loss or destruction of vitamins may not be due, or not due entirely, to heat.

Emmett and Luros (1919) found that considerable degrees of temperature did not affect the growth promoting value of lact-albumin.

Steenbock and Boutwell (1920) found from their experimental results that a process of heat treatment consisting of autoclaving for three hours at 15 lbs. pressure does not destroy any of the fat soluble vitamin as found in yellow maize. Neither does this treatment cause any noticeable destruction of the vitamin in carrots, sweet potato and other vegetables when these materials are fed in percentages of the ration varying from 5 to 15. They add: "our experiments demonstrate that the fat soluble vitamin as found in the plant kingdom in a grain, in leaf and stem tissue, in fleshy roots and in cucurbitous vegetable, is comparatively stable at a high temperature."

An experiment recorded by Professor Hopkins (1920) probably furnishes one clue to these discrepant results. Two groups of rats were fed, one set with butter which had been heated for four hours to 120° C. but heated without aeration, the other set with the same butter heated in exactly the same way but during the heating a stream of air was bubbled through the melted fat. In the first set there was normal growth, in the second definite weight loss, ill health and death. He remarks: "the results show definitely that oxidation plays a much larger part in the conditions which destroy than does temperature."

In a more detailed account of these experiments Hopkins (1920) showed that while four hours' exposure to 120° C. does not, in the absence of air, appreciably reduce the vitamin content of butter, aeration for four hours and even two hours at that temperature destroys most if not all the vitamin. Even one hour's aeration produced material destruction. Exposure of butter at ordinary temperature (15–25° C.) to air in thin layers for about a week was found to be adequate to destroy this vitamin.

Drummond and Coward (1920) also found that this vitamin in butter fat was rapidly destroyed on heating in the presence of air and that this may occur, if air exposure is extensive, at temperatures as low as 37° C.

Drummond, Coward and Watson (1920) concluded that the storage of butter and its preservation by such methods as tinning do not appear to lower the vitamin A value unless changes of an oxidative character take place.

As regards condensed milks McCollum (personal communication) has carried out some direct experiments. Using fats separated from different condensed milks he found (with one exception) they were capable equally with unheated fats of restoring the rats on a vitamin free diet to a healthy condition. The fats were from both sweetened and unsweetened milks.

Daniels and Stuessy (1916) observed that rats fed with milk boiled 1, 10, and 45 minutes respectively, grew slowly, failed to achieve the expected weight for normal animals and never reproduced. The authors suggest another explanation than loss of vitamin and this possibility is referred to below.

Barnes and Hume (1919) state that no significant difference was detected in the growth promoting properties of raw and dried milk respectively and this was true of both guinea-pigs and monkeys.

Water soluble B (anti-neuritic). This accessory factor is comparatively deficient in meat and milk and the tinned foods of chief importance which might contain it are the cereals (corn, peas, beans) and possibly some vegetables and fruits. The general experimental evidence is to the effect that this vitamin is rather thermolabile and as regards canned foods the M.R.C. report (1919, p. 34) states definitely: "In preserving and canning food stuffs, the temperatures employed are frequently much higher than 100° C. and it is safe to regard tinned foods of all descriptions with but few exceptions as vitamin free."

The investigations recorded do not all however confirm this conclusion.

Experiments by Chick and Hume (1917) may be summarized by saying that destruction of this vitamin takes place very slowly at 100° C. but is much more rapid in the neighbourhood of 120° C.

Miller (1920) on the other hand found that cooking carrots at 100° C. for 30 minutes caused no reduction in the vitamin, neither was there any destruction when carrots were lightly packed in a jar and heated at 125° C. for 45 minutes. Cooking navy beans at 120° C. for 30 minutes decreased the vitamin content 40 per cent. This worker and also Daniels and McClury found that a large proportion of the vitamin is found in the cooking water.

Johnson (1921) found that pasteurized milk and reconstructed milk made from milk dried by the spraying process had not lost their anti-neuritic vitamins.

Daniels and Loughlin (1920) investigated the vitamin content of both sweetened and unsweetened condensed milk. While the animals fed with unsweetened milk failed to grow and ultimately died, the growth curves of the animals fed with sweetened milk were fairly comparable to those of normal animals. By further experiments they arrived at the opinion that this was not due to loss of vitamins either A or B but was due to chemical alterations in the constitution of the milk and a loss of calcium phosphate. With thickened heat-treated milk good results were obtained. Rats fed with super-heated milk, supplemented with calcium phosphate properly incorporated, made normal growth gains.

Anti-scorbutic vitamin. The heat stability of this vitamin is not high and it seems to be particularly influenced by the speed of heating.

Campbell and Chick (1919) state definitely "In the process of canning vegetables the greater part of the original anti-scurvy value of the raw vegetable is destroyed. In the case of runner pod beans the loss is estimated at about 90 per cent. of the original value; in the case of cabbages it is about 70 per cent. of the original value. The process of canning cabbage included heating in water for about one hour at 90° C. to 100° C. and for beans the process was repeated on the day following."

Hart, Steenbock and Smith (1919) found that milk sterilized at 120° C. for 10 minutes had lost its scorbutic protective powers. Working with two brands of un-sweetened condensed milk they found that both had lost their anti-scorbutic properties. Hess and Ungar found that milk does not lose its anti-scorbutic properties to any extent if dried quickly.

Barnes and Hume (1919) found milk to be compara-tively poor in anti-scorbutic properties and that dried milk had lost about half its anti-scorbutic value.

Hess and Unger (1918) found that 5 c.c. of canned tomatoes was sufficient to protect guinea-pigs, kept on a diet which normally would lead to the development of scurvy, from developing that disease, while larger amounts stimulated growth to a remarkable degree. They recommend canned tomatoes for infant feeding as an economical and efficient anti-scorbutic.

Delf (1920) carried out experiments with the juice of oranges which had been canned and stored at laboratory temperatures for 5 months. The canning process in-volved heating in closed cans for 20–30 minutes, the temperature gradually rising from about 80° to 100° C. and remaining at the higher temperature for not more than five minutes. 1·5 c.c. daily of the fresh juice was still found to protect experimental animals from scurvy, the same dose as was required with fresh orange juice. Heating to 130° C. diminished the anti-scorbutic value and 3 c.c. was the daily dose necessary to give protec-tion. The heating was in the absence of air.

Hume (1921) using monkeys found that with two batches of sweetened condensed milk there was no definite loss of anti-scorbutic vitamin as compared with unprepared milk. There was also no appreciable loss of Vitamin A.

Jephcott and Bacharach (1921) found little or no impairment of anti-scorbutic value in dried milk as compared with fresh milk.

Zilva (1922) found that two hours' boiling did not destroy the anti-scorbutic potency of decitrated lemon juice in an atmosphere of carbon dioxide, whereas one hour's boiling in the presence of air destroyed its potency almost entirely.

Tinned meats and other preserved foods can be accepted as having little or no anti-scorbutic properties. The only exception of importance appears to be canned tomatoes and possibly other canned fruits.

The facts mentioned above show that it is not possible to give a simple direct answer to the question as to whether vitamins are present in canned foods. Very many factors are concerned. We have to remember that the whole of our knowledge as to vitamins is quite recent, that these substances are present in only minute quantities, that they have never been isolated in a pure state, that the only methods available for their detection require considerable experience if judgment is to be sound and are liable to many fallacies.

We have in addition to remember that the methods of preparation of foods by canning are both complicated and variable and the changes induced may be considerable and are much more than merely the effect of the application of a particular degree of heat. In other words we have to take into consideration not only the degree of heat applied to the product but also its method and particularly its rate of application. The chemical changes cannot be ignored, such as changes in hydrogen-ion concentration, oxidation, or colloidal changes. The factor of time since canning may be important since these vitamins are affected by storage and canned foods may be kept for years. Finally the quantitative factor is of essential importance and the fact that sufficient vitamins may be left to prevent pathological effects does not prove that they may not be dangerously diminished.

With all these variable and uncertain factors affecting the result, it is imperative that great caution be exercised in stating that any canned foods retain unimpaired the vitamins which they contained in the raw state.

With our present knowledge it is a reasonable attitude to take up that the whole complex of changes which are necessary in canning foods are detrimental to their content in vitamins, that these changes are more marked the greater the manipulation generally but are especially affected by the oxidation allowed and the temperatures reached in processing. Of temperature influences the three most potent are the actual temperature reached, the time given at that temperature, and the rapidity with which it is attained.

It is further evident that the three types of vitamins which are at present recognized are not equally affected by these adverse influences. The A type is comparatively heat stable and if the heat applied is not too high, is quickly applied and is not maintained for long, there may be no material diminution in the vitamin content. In actual practical conditions it has been found that these conditions are often fulfilled so that experimental results have shown comparatively slight reduction in this vitamin.

As regards the B type the evidence is that this is more thermolabile, and with any considerable application of heat it is likely to be entirely destroyed or dangerously reduced. We do not yet know, however, how far this is influenced by oxidation, and Professor Hopkins, who was kind enough to look over these notes, tells me that when oxygen is rigorously excluded this vitamin also shows a very considerable resistance to heat.

Vitamin C is still less resistant to heat and it is probably safe to assume that it is nearly completely absent in most canned foods.

GENERAL CONCLUSIONS

From the above detailed consideration of the different factors which may cause canned foods to be prejudicial to health clearly emerges the general conclusion that while they have definite and special risks of their own these are not large and are for the most part readily guarded against. Compared with fresh foods and the very haphazard, inadequate and neglected control which they receive canned foods are undoubtedly safer. They should not be made the main articles of diet, and provided this is avoided any possible deficiency of vitamins is readily made good from other sources. Experience and direct study have alike shown that the danger from tin poisoning is negligible. In relation to food poisoning outbreaks they take their share but not, according to my figures, an undue share as vehicles of infection. The special liability to cause botulism poisoning is serious on account of the fatality when it does occur but insignificant in its incidence. The risk of Salmonella poisoning from their consumption is one which cannot be regarded lightly, as probably many cases due to toxin poisoning are not recorded. The elimination of this risk is part of the general problem of the suppression of food poisoning and is dependent on a greater control of sources of infection. It is very necessary that steps should be taken in the places of origin of these meat and marine canned food products to recognize and eliminate infection of the food with Salmonella strains before canning. The harmfulness of these toxin and living bacillus outbreaks to the trade is very great and neither its danger nor the possibility of its removal is at all adequately realized.

The problem of spoilage is directly related to health considerations not to any material degree because spoiled canned foods are likely to cause illness, since this toxicity is slight and the risk of their consumption small, but mainly because the proportion of spoilage directly affects the question of price. Cheap pure food is one of the most potent factors in improving the health of the community and anything which increases the cost of canned foods is a health consideration.

The extension of the use of canned foods can only be advocated from the public health point of view if we can be satisfied, not only that the quality is sound but that the price per 1000 calories or other unit compares reasonably, and after due allowance for saving in fuel etc., with the cost of a similar unit of the fresh food. Amongst the poorer classes the money available for food frequently does not allow more than a bare minimum standard of nutrition to be attained, and to divert any considerable proportion of that money to canned foods yielding less energy per unit for the same expenditure may have a disastrous effect on the health of the community. It is for this reason amongst others that spoilage problems have been dealt with at length in Lecture II and considered to be germane to lectures devoted to canned food in relation to health.

In different sections of these lectures the defects which still exist in the preparation of these foods and in the methods of their distribution have been pointed out. The improvements in recent years have been material but there should be no slackening in endeavour by the trade itself and by pressure from outside to rectify these defects which are neither considerable nor difficult to remove. Their elimination is likely to extend still more their use.

No one who has studied the subject can be left in doubt as to the very great value of this method of preservation to the community. It enables large quantities of food to be utilized which otherwise would be wasted, no mean Public Health advantage. Any dangers from their use are not great and are at least as easily controllable as from the use of unprepared foods.

APPENDIX I

NOTES ON THE PRINCIPLES INVOLVED IN THE PROCESSING OF CANNED FOODS

By WILLIAM G. SAVAGE

Reprinted with the permission of the Food Investigation Board.

THE expression "processing" is the technical term applied in the trade to the final heating given to the product in the can after it has been hermetically sealed, and is designed to render the product safe from subsequent bacterial decomposition. The word "sterilization" is sometimes employed as its equivalent but is an unsatisfactory term since it implies something definite, i.e. that the product has been rendered free from living bacteria, an implication which is not in accordance with the facts. The word "processing" commits one to nothing and is therefore preferable.

In processing operations there are two objectives:

(*a*) To subject the canned foods to a degree of heat which will either actually sterilize the product or which will at least kill out all forms which may subsequently develop and cause spoilage or illness when the food is consumed.

(*b*) The degree and duration of the heat treatment must be such as will not damage the food-stuff as a commercial product.

Commercial considerations necessitate that the second objective must be complied with, so that in actual practice the degree of heating given under the first condition is conditioned by and subordinate to the second. The problem of the practical canner is not therefore to ascertain the temperature conditions which the expert points out, or his practical experience indicates, as adequate to ensure sterility and then apply them to his products, but the more delicate one of the application of the degree of heat which he knows will not injure his product and yet will ensure a very high percentage of tins which will remain sound as judged by commercial and practical standards.

The details of the problem are not the same for all foods since both the resistance to heat of the bacteria present and the liability to damage of the food canned vary with each product. In some instances his margin of safety is a wide one and his problem easy of solution, in others the critical margin is narrow. Unsweetened condensed milk is a good example of a food with a narrow margin of safety. Spore resistant bacterial strains are liable to be present which require a high temperature, often a sustained high temperature, to kill, while on the other hand this food is very liable to be damaged as a commercial product from the application of heat at a high temperature. In such a case it is necessary to study with great care the factors which influence the problem and to conduct the processing with a nice regard to accuracy.

In the same connection it may be mentioned that with some fruits heating to about 100° C. injures their appearance and flavour so that with these fruits the tendency is to keep the temperature low and secure bacterial destruction by prolonging the time of exposure.

These preliminary remarks will make clear how very necessary it is to study with considerable care and detail the different factors which affect the application of heat to canned foods.

These factors can conveniently be discussed under three headings, i.e. the bacteria present, the character and composition of the food in the can, and technical and physical points affecting the temperature required.

A. The bacteria present or possibly present

From the point of view of their resistance to heat bacteria fall into three groups:

1. Bacteria which form spores.
2. The ordinary non-sporing type of bacillus.
3. Certain more resistant non-sporing types. Of these the most important are the tubercle bacillus and some types of streptococci.

From the standpoint of the canner the only classes of any importance and interest are those which are pathogenic and those which cause spoilage.

Fortunately the only type of sporing bacillus pathogenic to man which may be present in canned food is *B. botulinus*. *B. anthracis* is theoretically possible but may be ignored in practice. Most of the pathogenic bacteria are of low resistance and do not require special consideration. The possibility of survival of pathogenic streptococci and *B. tuberculosis* almost entirely concerns milk products and is discussed in the special reports on those foods.

Of considerable importance is the question of the survival of heat-resisting toxins of the Salmonella group and possibly of *B. botulinus*. These important matters are discussed in detail elsewhere. They are all rare contingencies which have to be guarded against rather by means which prevent access of the bacilli than by any special temperatures of processing. In actual cannery practice the problem which is dominant is that of eliminating the bacteria which may cause spoilage.

In addition to the resistance to heat of the types of bacteria the initial numbers present when the stage of processing is reached have to be taken into account.

The number of bacteria present is of great importance. It is well established that the rate of destruction of bacteria by heat varies with the number of bacteria. As H. Chick (1910) has shown, disinfection may be considered analogous to a chemical reaction the velocity of which is controlled by external conditions, including temperature and concentration of the bacteria. Disinfection proceeds in accordance with a logarithmic law so that the concentration of survivors varies logarithmically with time. In other words, the rate of disinfection at any moment is proportional to the concentration of surviving bacteria. This has been stated mathematically as regards the death of bacteria when subjected to any fixed unfavourable conditions, i.e.

$$k = \frac{1}{t} \log \frac{B}{b},$$

where k = velocity coefficient of the rate of death of bacteria—a constant,
t = interval of time between observations,
B = number of bacteria at beginning of any time interval,
b = number of bacteria at end of time t.

The number of living bacteria present at the time of processing is a factor of considerable importance in relation to spoilage. It emphasises the need for cleanliness conditions in the preliminary stages and throughout the manufacturing processes. Some products such as tomatoes are liable to be heavily contaminated with soil and they have to receive very thorough washing before they can be utilized, otherwise soil bacteria, many being highly resistant sporing types, may be retained alive in the product when it goes into the processing retorts. In my experience with a fish such as herrings, which frequently has tomato sauce added as an adjuvant, a higher proportion of tins are found non-sterile when this sauce is used than when no adjuvant or some other sauce is employed.

In the report on the Bacteriology of meat and marine products the importance of avoiding canning sardines which had just fed was pointed out, since they were liable to be heavily contaminated with bacteria and in practice considerable trouble is taken to keep them in water pens until they are empty of feed. Here the difficulty of sterilizing a food product containing many bacteria is recognized.

Bigelow and Esty (*vide infra*), working under practical conditions with the spores of thermophilic bacteria in corn juice, give figures they obtained illustrating the importance of the numerical factor. The following may be quoted:

Strain	Initial concentration of spores	Minutes required to destroy spores at 115° C.
26	45,000 400 40	65 28 22
1890	35,000 275 58	42 21 10
1390	70,000 600 65	42 23 13

It is undoubtedly of great importance in successful canning, i.e., to obtain a very small percentage of spoilage, to obtain the food as clean and bacterially free as possible and to pass it through the different preparation stages so that multiplication of bacteria does not occur to any material extent.

The importance of the relationship between time and temperature is universally recognized but has recently been studied as regards its relationship to canned foods by Bigelow and Esty (1920). They worked with resistant spore-bearing thermophilic bacteria, all recently isolated from canned foods, and tested their heat resistance suspended in juices of canned foods (corn, peas, string beans, beets, etc.) of an accurately determined hydrogen-ion concentration. As regards this particular point their results show how important is this relationship. For example, 200,000 spores per c.c. of their culture No. 26 were destroyed in 13,200 minutes at 100° C., in 690 minutes at 105° C., in 225 minutes at 110° C., in 84 minutes at 115° C., in 23 minutes at 120° C., in 8 minutes at 135° C., and in 1 minute at 140° C. Nineteen thermophilic organisms showed a very similar relationship between time and temperature.

They also noted the point, which is well recognized as regards bacteria generally, that spores of the same organism varied in resistance to heat under special conditions and that this resistance could be increased greatly. For example, one type was increased from a time of 12 to 23 minutes to kill at 120° C. within six months through repeated artificial cultivation. Also by careful selection of surviving spores a very resistant type was produced.

B. THE INFLUENCE OF THE CHARACTER AND COMPOSITION OF THE FOOD IN THE CAN

These, although varied, can be grouped into three classes:

(1) The physical properties of the food as affecting heat transference.

(2) The acidity or, more accurately, the hydrogen-ion concentration of the food.

(3) The protective properties of the contents as affecting the resistance of the bacteria.

(1) The physical properties of the food. The character of the food in the can is of fundamental importance. Heat is for the most part conducted into the centre of cans by conduction and convection. Convection currents are markedly affected by the nature of the food.

When the food inside the can is solid or nearly solid the penetration of heat is almost entirely by conduction and therefore penetration is relatively slow. When a solid is mixed with water as the fluid, convection currents are freely formed and we get rapid heat penetration and the rate is not materially impaired when salt solution or dilute syrup replaces the water. Starch on the other hand greatly impedes the formation of convection currents and greatly retards heat penetration.

The subject has recently been studied by Bigelow and his co-workers (1920) in special relationship to canned foods, and the following remarks are largely taken from their valuable Bulletin. They have shown that when the percentage of starch is only 1–2 its effect is noticeable and becomes more marked as the amount of starch is increased until a 5 to 6 per cent. solution is reached. No further retardation takes place above six per cent., showing that above this percentage heat penetration is almost entirely due to conduction alone. Conduction itself is however affected by rising temperature.

Starch is a colloid and it is probable that other colloids will behave similarly. The same point arises in regard to unsweetened condensed milk. To mention an example from my own experience, in one experiment with a tin of unsweetened milk at an initial temperature of 18° C. immersed in boiling water it took 35 minutes for the thermometer in the centre to reach 90° C., while when raw milk was substituted it took only six minutes and distilled water only three minutes.

Products which alter when heated so that they pack together and products that are cooked to pieces during the process make the contents somewhat viscous and retard heat penetration. Bitting (1916) points out that fruit packers have experienced greater losses in packing over-ripe stock than in packing that which is green and that this is due to the fact that the very soft ripe stock tends to mat together and prevent the liquid from circulating between the pieces, diminishing convection currents. A similar condition occurs in canning very ripe tomatoes, especially if heavy *purée* is added to fill the interstices.

The size of the particles is of some influence. Heat takes time to penetrate so that large particles are as a whole at a lower temperature than the liquid surrounding them and they exert a cooling influence upon it.

The slow rate of heat penetration into canned meat was shown long ago by Beveridge and Fawcus (1908). They also found the rate of penetration to be very variable.

Bigelow and his co-workers (1920) extensively studied the application of these laws to practical canning conditions, recording a long series of observations. They used a special form of thermocouple capable of being used to test the processing of canned foods under actual factory conditions. Using a number of leads they were able to take a number of simultaneous observations. A stuffing box was soldered to the top of the can to introduce the thermocouple. To get accurate results it is essential that the joint should be tight and this was obtained by the use of a rubber gasket. The measurement of the voltage of the electric current generated from the difference of temperature between the joints of two wires soldered together enables the temperature to be calculated, one joint of course being kept at a known temperature. In their Bulletin the results obtained are plotted in the form of graphs, the horizontal lines showing the temperatures reached, the vertical the number of minutes taken to reach the temperature indicated. The temperatures recorded were at the centre of the can. The different curves obtained deserve careful study and show that the rate of heat penetration to the centre is affected by different kinds and qualities of the content, even of the same food product. For example, with salmon when it is packed solid, heat penetration is very slow but with smaller pieces surrounded by some liquid the heat penetration rate is considerably increased. With plums heat penetration to the centre of the can is slower than with peas, because the plums are larger. This retardation is materially increased if a heavy syrup is used instead of water, and the curves obtained show that with a 50 per cent. syrup they may take over twice as long (45 minutes instead of 20 minutes) to reach retort temperature.

Bovie and Bronfenbrenner (1919) have also described an apparatus for measuring the rate of heat penetration which is a thermocouple of rather different construction.

G. E. Thompson (1919) has also determined by means of thermocouples the temperature-time curves at the centre of tins subjected to various temperatures. He makes the same point as the other observers, that substances which contain a great deal of free liquid heat up almost as fast as water if the liquid is of low viscosity but increase of viscosity markedly retards. He draws attention to the influence of the change of viscosity with temperature. His paper is essentially on mathematical lines.

The mathematical side of the problem, including a formula to calculate the temperature at the centre of the can, is further discussed by Buchanan, Thompson, Orr and Bennett (1918). They set out a formula which they found to be applicable generally except at the beginning of the heating. They found that their theoretical and experimental curves showed close agreement, both in heating and in cooling.

(2) The acidity and hydrogen-ion concentration of the food. The importance of the factor of acidity in relation to the destruction of bacteria has long been recognized. For example, H. Chick (1910) testing the rate of destruction by heat of *B. typhosus* in broth found the rate to be much slower in broth than in distilled water. This was found to be due to the slight alkalinity of the broth. The addition of a small extra amount of acid, too small to exert any disinfection action of itself, rendered disinfection so quick that the rate could not be measured and the velocity constant of disinfection was more than 40 times as great as in the original broth.

Bigelow and Esty (1920) working with very resistant spores suspended in different vegetable juices found that the time necessary for their destruction was materially affected by this factor. With a known number of spores at a given temperature they found that as the P_H value is increased the time required for complete destruction is decreased. The authors did not vary the P_H value with the same juice but they believe that the time necessary to destroy spores with the other factors constant (temperature, number of spores, etc.) varies with the different juices just so far as these P_H values are different.

In a later Bulletin, Bigelow and Cathcart (1921) further discuss this relationship and give figures showing the range of P_H values of most canned foods. They found considerable differences in the contents of individual cans. They also note that the heat of processing causes a decrease in the P_H value in most cases. This they suggest may be due partially to an actual production of acids and partially by a precipitation of buffer substances.

(3) **The protective properties of the contents as affecting the resistance of the bacteria.** There are two ways in which an influence may be exerted. In the first place it must be borne in mind that estimations as to the time required to kill bacteria in canned food products are largely based, for most foods, upon the time required to kill surface bacteria. Put another way, experiments recorded as to temperatures reached in the interior of cans are temperatures reached by liquids in the centre. For foods such as fruits or vegetables they are not the temperatures of the centre of such fruits. For more or less uniform liquids such as milk or closely packed foods such as canned meats this point does not arise but it does for other foods. Probably it is most important as regards canned fish and other marine products. The temperatures reached may be adequate to kill all surface bacteria but they may be insufficient to enable a lethal temperature to be reached

by the centre of the fish. The point has already been mentioned as regards the importance of only canning sardines freed from feed. These fish are not gutted and if *B. coli* and other gas producing bacilli are in the intestinal contents in any numbers they may be protected from destruction by the fish tissues surrounding them, the heat of the interior of the fish being sub-lethal. Fortunately with most canned products the bacteria are all on or near the surface and the interior is sterile. With meat on the other hand the pieces are broken up quite small and the immersion in the pickling fluid introduces living bacteria right through much of the food. The cooking and processing given have therefore to be adequate to raise all parts to a temperature fatal to bacterial life, if sterility is to be reached.

The other protective influence is more problematical; with substances such as milk the bacteria may be protected to some extent by being enveloped in the fat or albuminous constituents and so be more resistant to heat. Very little, however, is known on this point. The well attested increased difficulty of destroying bacteria in milk as compared to water may be merely a physical question of the difference of heat conduction through the mass.

C. TECHNICAL AND PHYSICAL POINTS AFFECTING THE TEMPERATURE REQUIRED

There is a number of points closely related to practical canning operations which have to be kept in mind in considering the temperatures used in processing which have not yet been considered but which are of material importance. The following are the most important:

1. **The size of the containers used.** It is self-evident that large cans will require a longer time at the same temperature for the centre to reach the same degree of

heat. Cans of larger size are always processed for a longer time than those of smaller size. Bigelow (1920) states that for cans longer than their diameter the time necessary for heat to penetrate to the centre of the can is approximately proportional to the square of the radius of the can. Williamson and Adams (1919) and also Thompson (1918) have published equations and calculations which make it possible to calculate the theoretical heat penetration curves in canned foods and these include the size of the container.

Calculations of this kind are more applicable to products of slow heat penetration than to those in which convection currents play a material share in heat transfer.

2. Influence of the initial temperature. With products such as peas and many fruits, where heat passes rapidly to the centre of the can, this factor is not very important, but with products in which heat penetration is slow the initial temperature is of great importance. With food of this nature the processing should be done as quickly as possible after the tins are filled and sealed, i.e. before they have had time to cool down. In most canning operations the contents of the can are heated up before the can is sealed, as this gives a vacuum.

3. Form in which the heat is applied. While the source of heat is steam, it may be applied as dry steam or as a mixture of water and steam. Bigelow (1920) studied this point experimentally and remarks "so far as we have been able to determine, there is no difference in the rapidity of heat penetration, whether processing in dry steam or under water." He points out, however, that in the technique of various canning plant there are differences in detail which greatly influence the results. For instance, while in some plants the retorts are partially or entirely filled with water which is heated practically to the boiling point before the tins are introduced, in others the tins are put into the water when it is comparatively cold which is then gradually heated while the other crates of tins are being filled in. In the latter procedure the tins are actually cooled first. These points really illustrate the influence of the initial temperature rather than the form of heat.

4. **Influence of rotation of the cans.** It is obvious that heat penetration is materially influenced by agitation of the contents so that within recent years considerable attention has been paid to the development of agitating cookers. The usual plan is for the interior framework to revolve so that the cans are rotated.

Rotation is of considerably greater value for some products than for others. It is least beneficial for foods which are packed dry, which have a heavy consistency or which tend to move *en masse* when the can is rotated (Bitting). Or as Bigelow puts it, dealing with agitating cookers, "They are of value in processing products which at sterilizing temperatures are sufficiently fluid to permit them to mix readily but which do not permit the free movement of convection currents."

Bitting (1916) states that the greatest advantage from the use of the agitating cooker is not so much in the shortening of the time of cooking as in the possibility of lowering the temperature and thereby gaining in quality. "The time of cooking for most products is reduced to about one-fourth that necessary for the same product when standing, and it has been reduced on some products like tomatoes to one-tenth the regular cooking period."

Violent agitation is not required; the aim is to allow the solids to shift so that the liquid portions may move through the mass.

5. **Influence of subsequent cooling upon sterilization.** It is obvious that if the canned products are cooled quickly after the processing any sterilizing heat effects are cut off more rapidly than if the products cool slowly and are allowed to remain at high temperatures

for a considerable time. Any such action is, however, very uncertain and irregular and the disadvantages are far greater than any additional bactericidal action. In practice therefore it is the usual procedure to employ some form of rapid cooling immediately after processing. Any additional sterilizing effects should not be relied upon or employed. Incidentally it may be mentioned, as bearing upon the temperature of processing, that the sudden cooling throws a great strain upon the cans. The higher the temperature of processing the greater the strain. Its greatest severity is exerted when the hot cans are suddenly subjected to cold water. Commonly the cans are partially cooled in the retorts by running in cold water and again cooled outside the retorts by cold water applied as a jet or by immersion in it.

General Observations

The very large number of factors which affect the temperatures and times required for absolute sterilization shows how complicated is the whole matter and how impracticable it is to set down precise data in regard to these two factors which shall be generally applicable. It is only within the last few years that any serious attempt has been made to remove the subject from one of empiricism to one on a scientific basis, and in spite of the valuable results which have been achieved very much remains to be done. The facts mentioned, and also practical experience, show that while rule of thumb procedures may yield satisfactory results, on many occasions untoward results are apt to occur unaccountably from time to time and often resulting from what appear to be trifling matters.

The bacteriological reports which we have furnished show how large is the number of perfectly sound samples which contain living bacteria, or in other words for a large proportion of canned food tins processing is not identical with sterilization. These results further show that the criterion of absolute sterility may not be of material moment and that, for example, killing vegetable forms may be as efficient as the employment of temperatures which kill the spores also, since under many conditions the latter are incapable of reproduction. It is probably this fact and this safeguard, rather than any absolute sterility efficiency of the processing which has enabled so many empirically devised processing procedures to give satisfactory results.

Until the influence of the various factors indicated above has been accurately worked out we are a long way from being able to prescribe exact times and temperatures for processing which can be relied upon to give uniformly satisfactory results and yet not injure the contents.

APPENDIX II

REPORT UPON LABORATORY METHODS FOR THE EXAMINATION OF CANNED FOODS

By William G. Savage

Reprinted with the permission of the Food Investigation Board.

In view of the very extensive importation of canned foods into this country the trifling attention which has been given to Laboratory methods of examination is rather remarkable. Little or nothing has been contributed to this subject in Great Britain. On the other hand, as might be anticipated from the extensive nature of the canned food industry in the United States of America, considerable work has been done in that country although there still remains a good deal to be accomplished. In the present report this work is extensively utilized both as set out in published papers and more particularly from practical experience in America. The writer is particularly indebted to Dr W. D. Bigelow, Chief Chemist, National Canners' Association, for placing at his disposal his ripe experience in these matters and for his practical demonstrations at the well-equipped laboratories at Washington of the National Canners' Association.

In addition the writer with his associate workers has been continuously engaged for over three years in a systematic study of canned food during which over 800 tins of different canned foods were exhaustively studied. This has afforded extensive experience as regards many of these methods, while special procedures have been devised to meet some of the difficulties encountered and to enable a more accurate judgment to be given as to the condition of the containers and their contents. Many thousands of tins have also been examined at the ports of entry.

Section A. Examination of the container

The methods of examination employed by the Food Inspectors have been described in other reports. The present report is only concerned with examinations in the Laboratory.

1. **Types of can.** While shapes and sizes vary widely, practically all the tins used in commercial canning conform to one of two types—"Hole and cap" and the "Sanitary." The former is the original type but is being rapidly supplanted by the "Sanitary" can, since the latter is more readily filled and closed and, although it is not cheaper to make, its filling and closing is more economical so that it is regarded as a cheaper package for the canner.

As the name suggests the hole and cap tins have a fairly large circular opening at the top to admit the food. When filled this is covered by a cap, the margins of which overlap the edge of the hole. When ready for sealing the margins are soldered down, the solder usually being already coated over the edge of the cap to facilitate the operation.

The centre of the cap has a small hole to allow the heated expanded air to escape, otherwise the soldering might be troublesome, and this is finally closed by a dab of solder. The tins have the advantage that the joints of cap and tin can be made sound and air tight without much difficulty. There is some small risk of lead from solder entering the can but this is trifling and the danger of lead poisoning nearly negligible.

In the sanitary type of can the top is open. After filling, the lid is laid on the top and by means of a special machine is crimped on by double seaming. No solder is used in this operation and the only solder in the tin is that used in making tight the single side seam. To ensure air tightness a gasket is used. This is often in the form of a previously painted on ring of a solution containing rubber, but a paper gasket is a frequently used contrivance. In tins, such as for sardines, where no gasket is used the double seam cannot be relied upon to ensure air exclusion but the oil may prevent air leakage.

The interior of the containers may be plain or lacquered. Lacquering of the tins is done for two purposes, the chief being for trade purposes to preserve colour and appearance, the other to prevent or diminish the action of any acid food product upon the metal of the container. The use of paper or parchment linings for products such as crabs and lobsters is also for trade purposes, i.e. to prevent discoloration of the food.

2. External appearance. This has been described in other reports. The presence of extensive rust is of considerable significance since it means denudation of the metal which later will result in actual perforation. Rusty places should be very carefully cleaned and the places scrutinized very closely for actual leaks.

The presence of vent holes must be carefully noted but their presence may be perfectly legitimate and no evidence of the venting and re-closure of an unsound tin. (See Special Report No. 3 Food Investigation Board, Methods used for the Inspection of Canned Meats.)

3. Examination for a vacuum. The outline of methods of manufacture which has been given in the different reports will make it evident that for most foods a definite vacuum should be present. The amount of any vacuum will, however, vary greatly not only with different products but with the same class of product. With meat foods a considerable vacuum is almost invariably obtained. Some vacuum is usually present with canned marine products and fruit but with some foods such as sardines it is usually very slight, in our experience. On the other hand we have usually found but little vacuum with unsweetened condensed milk although perfectly sound and for the most part no vacuum at all, or none we could detect, with sweetened condensed milk. With the latter product little or no attempt is made to make the cans air tight. While the absence of a vacuum cannot be taken as in any way a ground for rejection (although with many products it suggests a leak), its presence is of great importance. It is direct evidence of the absence of any leak, even a microscopic leak, and a reliable guide proving the absence of patency of the container.

It can be readily ascertained with a vacuum gauge of special type. The gauge ends in a stout hollow needle the cavity of which is in continuity with the gauge and the end of which is sharpened. Over the needle is a good quality rubber cork. The tin is punctured, the rubber being well pressed at the time of puncture against the surface of the tin. This makes an air-tight joint and any vacuum is at once read off on the gauge.

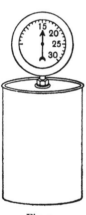

Fig. 1.

The procedure is very simple and the only difficulty is the unfortunate facility with which the needle becomes choked. The accuracy of the gauge should be tested from time to time.

4. **Detection of leaks.** Our investigations have impressed us very strongly with the importance of leaks as a potent cause of unsoundness, not because they admit bacteria, but because they allow the access of air. The admission of oxygen enables bacteria already present, but dormant, to resume their activities and spoil the product.

The detection of leaks is therefore of considerable importance.

Several methods are available.

(*a*) **Direct examination.** While large leaks are obvious on careful inspection, it is very difficult and often impossible to detect minute leaks by simple naked eye examination. With foods such as fruits, with partially liquid contents, their detection is assisted by violently knocking the tin on some hard surface. This also may unseal small leaks blocked up by dirt or food particles but it is only the more crude leaks which can be detected in this way. Occasionally placing in hot water, which dissolves fat and gelatine which may plug a leak, and squeezing under the water may show a leak by the extrusion of a bubble of air, but we have not found this procedure of much service.

Even with a tin, which from other parts of the examination is known to be leaky, or in which a leak is subsequently detected by one of the methods mentioned below, which has its contents emptied out and the paint washed off with dilute caustic potash it is often impossible to detect a leak by naked eye examination.

(*b*) **Water vacuum test.** This is a simple method which is sometimes successful but the facility with which particles of the contents block up the leaks militates greatly against its practical utility. The procedure is readily seen from the sketch. The tin is completely submerged in recently boiled water in a glass vessel with an air-tight lid with ground joint well luted.

The flat lid is perforated to take a tube connected with a vacuum pump and gauge (Fig. 2). Of course everything must be perfectly air tight. If the can leaks, operating the vacuum pump will cause bubbles to escape from the tin and rise through the water.

(*c*) **Testing for leaks under pressure.** This is the most reliable method but is somewhat troublesome. As practised at the National Canned Food Laboratory in

Washington in 1919 it was carried out as follows and
Dr Bigelow writes me in 1922 that this is the present
procedure.

By means of a tin opener a circular piece is cut out
of the top of the can about 1½ to 2 inches in diameter.
To obtain a circular opening one of the types of tin
opener which cuts a circular hole should be used. The
size of the hole should be slightly smaller than one of
the stock cap sizes. The contents (after any bacteriological examination) are removed. The tin is then

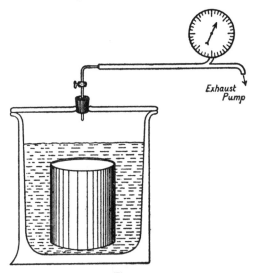

*Exhaust
Pump*

Fig. 2.

washed out thoroughly and boiled in ordinary water
for some time. All the water, as far as possible, is
sucked out and the tin is dried at 80° C. for an hour or
so. If it has a *paper* gasket this should not be done
since these tins are not warranted to be perfectly air
tight when completely dry. One of the stock tin covers,
which can be purchased with affixed solder rim, is then
placed over the hole and soldered on. It is convenient
and expeditious, but not essential, to use the special

circular soldering iron which is used commercially for
soldering hole and cap tins. The top must be held down
until the solder is quite hard. A careful examination
must be made to see that the joint is satisfactory. The
tin is now turned upside down and into the opposite
flat surface the special puncturing end of the apparatus
used (see Fig. 3) is inserted, rotated through a quarter
of a circle and the level pressed up to expand the india-
rubber ring at the junction and make an air-tight joint.
The whole apparatus is then placed in water sufficient
to completely cover the tin and junction and air is

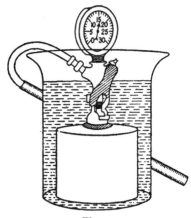

Fig. 3.

pumped in. At Washington this is done by connecting
to the air pump apparatus, but in my laboratory I use
an ordinary bicycle pump and this is quite satisfactory.
The tin is tested by gradual additions of 5 lbs. pressure,
read off on the gauge. Leaks are very obvious by the
escape of bubbles of air through the water.

The following pressures as standards are used :

No. 1 and No. 2 sized cans ... Tested by 5 lbs. pressure additions up to
25 lbs. pressure.

No. 2½ and No. 3 sized cans ... Tested by 5 lbs. pressure additions up to
15 lbs. pressure.

No. 10 sized can ... Tested by 5 lbs. pressure additions up to 10 lbs. pressure.

With leaks only showing at the very highest pressures one cannot be always certain that there was a leak originally in the tin as the test is a severe one. Even such a thorough procedure is not always sufficient to demonstrate leaks which have been thoroughly closed by particles of food.

In cases where the detection of a leak is not of primary importance and where time is of moment we have often been able to detect a leak by removing some of the contents for examination through a small hole and then using the same hole to perforate with the instrument. Air is then pumped in, the tin being under water, and the pressure is sufficient to force it through the contents through the leak. This obviates cleaning out and resoldering, but while valuable when positive evidence is obtained it is of little value as negative evidence of the absence of a leak.

5. **Examination of the construction of the can itself and the condition of the joints.** In a "sanitary" can the two chief points of weakness are the soldered joint forming the vertical seam down the side of the can and the crimped joint along which the lid is fixed to the receptacle.

The crimped joint is the more important since more likely to be defective. The lids are affixed by machines which have reached a high degree of efficiency and when properly adjusted the percentage of defective cans is an extremely small one. Like all machines they are emphatically not fool proof and require careful and daily adjustment by a skilled mechanic. This they do not always receive and in consequence a machine may be turning out a considerable percentage of inadequately closed cans. The following sketches (Fig. 4) illustrate properly closed seams and junctions which are defective.

The method employed to examine this crimped joint is to file away the tin along the line of the joint so as to expose the joint in section. The filings are cleaned

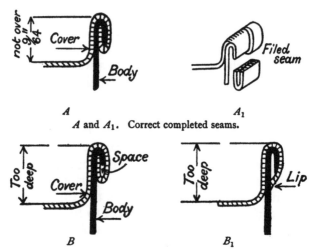

A and *A₁*. Correct completed seams.

B and *B₁*. Incorrect seam due to incorrect setting of machine.

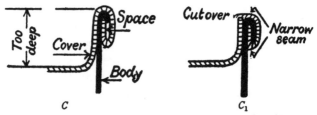

C and *C₁*. Incorrect seam due to incorrect setting of machine.

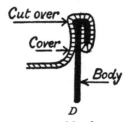

D. Incorrect seam resulting from worn chuck.

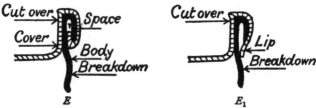

E and *E₁*. Incorrect seam from too much base pressure.

Fig. 4. Sanitary Can. Double Seams.

out with a pin and the cross section examined with a lens. It can then be readily seen if the crimping has been properly done or if one of the defects shown above is exhibited.

The actually weakest point in the whole can is the place of junction of the side seam with the crimped joint, so the place to start filing should be about an inch to the side of this point. By filing through the top curve of the crimped joint the lower piece is detached and it can then be seen if it is jointed properly at this weak junction.

The side seam of the can itself should then be stripped and carefully examined, with a lens if necessary, to see if it is perfectly soldered.

Incidentally it may be mentioned that the distinction between defects in these two joints is an important one practically to the trade. If the crimped joint on the lid side of the tin is defective it is due to imperfect work in the cannery, i.e. it is a fault which concerns the packer. If the defect is in any other joint, i.e. the side seam or the crimped edge at the bottom of the tin, it usually points to defective construction of the tins and so can properly be charged back to the makers of the cans.

With hole and cap cans the points of weakness are different. The chief places to look for leaks are the junctions of the cap, the central vent and leaks in the body seams, i.e. these may be cap leaks, vent leaks, body seam leaks. Cap leaks are due to defective soldering of the caps, the commonest cause being exudation of the contents which prevents the solder making a proper junction between the cap and the body of the tin. Vent leaks are in the solder filling the vent, and also may be due to particles of the food or juice preventing union. They are usually very minute and only the size of a hair and are then difficult to detect. Body leaks may be in any seam, top, bottom or side, and are due to defective tins and not to the sealing of the cans at the cannery.

Section B. Chemical analysis of the contents

This may be of two kinds, one for analytical purposes to judge the quality of the food, the other to estimate deviations of the food from the normal as a guide to unfitness. The former is purely a trade matter and outside the scope of this report. The latter may vary considerably with the nature of the food but broadly there are only five determinations which require mention.

1. **Determination of acidity.** While the estimation of the hydrogen-ion concentration is of material value in connection with canned foods it does not replace the simpler determination of titratable acidity. This is of considerable value and very readily carried out. It has been shown in the various reports that as a rule the variations of titratable acidity with the same food content are slight.

Any considerable deviations from these average figures therefore are of significance in judging the unfitness of the sample.

The determination is readily carried out by titration with $N/10$ alkali as described in a number of the Reports. With substances such as fruit, partially liquid partly solid, there is no need to take a mixture of the two and the titration of a definite quantity of the juice is easier and also more satisfactory. With solid substances, or mostly solid substances such as fish, definite weighed portions have to be taken.

2. **Examination for metals.** Tin, lead and occasionally iron have to be looked for. Satisfactory methods are given in the text-books.

3. **Analysis of the gas content.** This is chiefly used in connection with the examination of "blown" samples. While we have occasionally found it useful for research purposes to elucidate special points, there is but little to be gained by its utilization for the routine examination

of blown tins. A blown tin can safely be rejected however produced, and in practice, in spite of the theoretical
possibility of their production from chemical or physical
changes apart from bacterial activities, the condition is
almost invariably due to decomposition changes from
the activities of micro-organisms. It is a waste of time
to analyse the varieties of gases present.

On the other hand it should be mentioned that Dr
Bigelow and the American workers who are more closely
concerned with studies of factory conditions in relation
to spoilage than workers in this country find gas analysis
of considerable value.

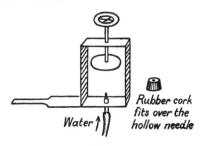

Fig. 5.

Since however it is useful occasionally to elucidate
obscure points of origin, the following method may be
mentioned.

The method and procedure described by Baker (*Report of the 8th International Congress of Applied
Chemistry*, 1912, Vol. XVIII. 43) and as explained personally to the writer gives satisfactory results.

As described by Baker the apparatus consists of an
extensible strap iron frame in which a can may be set
and clamped down by means of a screw clamp.

Entering at the base of this steel frame is a hollow
steel needle as shown in Fig. 5. The rubber stopper
shown alongside of this needle, in use, is placed over
the needle. It is of such height that the rubber stopper
must be considerably compressed before the needle

punctures the bottom of the can. The steel needle is connected with a water supply so that a stream of water under about 15 lbs. pressure can be forced through the puncturing needle into the can. Adequate water pressure from any source would be satisfactory.

The strap iron holder which is either screwed or clamped on to a table has a twisted iron shank so that it tips at an angle of approximately 45°. This clamp has a screw compression which works on the bottom of the can and a hollow steel puncturing needle through which the gas is extracted from the top of the can. The puncturing needle is enclosed in a rubber stopper so that compression and tight connection is necessary before the steel needle punctures the top of the can. The tilt places the can in such a position that it can be punctured and the gas drawn off into a Doremus or other Gas Extracting Apparatus from its highest point as shown in Fig. 6.

Any other kind of puncturing arrangement based on the same principle would answer satisfactorily.

The top of the gas extractor is connected with a gas burette by means of capillary tubing with rubber connections.

The complete procedure for extracting the gas is as follows:

After the can is in position, water is forced through the steel puncturing needle in the base and, while the water is still flowing through, the screw clamp from the top is turned down until the compression in the rubber stopper is great enough to allow the needle to puncture the base of the can. Water under pressure may then enter the can. The Doremus Clamp is then screwed down solidly, the hollow steel needle filled with water; the capillary connecting tubes between the gas burette and the extractor are filled with water and connected as shown in Fig. 6. The clamps on the rubber connections are then loosened, the gas burette opened and the

Doremus Clamp screwed down until the can is punctured. The gas then flows out through the capillary tubing, displacing the water in the gas burette.

When all the gas has been removed, some of the liquid in the can will come over and sweep any gas in the capillary connections into the gas burette so that quick and complete extraction of the gas from the headspace of the sample is obtained.

The gas analysis is conducted by ordinary methods. For canned goods the gases of importance are oxygen, nitrogen, carbon dioxide and hydrogen.

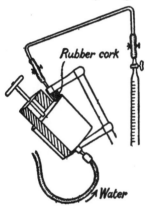

Fig. 6.

4. Examination for chemical signs of decomposition. It has been shown in another report[1] that it is a very difficult matter to determine the early stages of decomposition and to judge from naked eye appearances whether certain classes of canned foods, particularly marine products, are good or not. The advantage of chemical tests which can be applied at once has been explained in that report and also the fact that at present there are no reliable chemical criteria available. For a consideration of the tests which have been used reference should be made to that report.

[1] To be published shortly.

5. Examination for preservatives. Chemical preservatives are rarely found in canned foods at the present time. Such natural preservatives as sugar or salt are of course excluded from consideration. As Dr MacFadden showed in 1908 they were at one time common in potted and other prepared meat foods and should be looked for in such foods.

While they may be added to such preserved foods as jams or prepared meat foods there is usually no need to examine the ordinary tinned foods for preservatives except under special circumstances. The ordinary methods are applicable.

Section C. Bacteriological examination

This is discussed in detail in other reports and is only briefly mentioned here for completeness.

1. Examination of films made direct from the food and stained for micro-organisms. This is readily carried out and, as the reports on the different foods show, is of considerable value. It does not distinguish between the bacteria present which are living and those which are dead, but it does give a valuable insight into the conditions through which the food has passed before, during and after its introduction into the tin.

It is a simple procedure which should not be omitted.

2. Examination for living micro-organisms. In any comprehensive examination a considerable number of culture tubes must be inoculated since the varieties of bacteria, yeasts and moulds which may be present are numerous. Any examination purporting to be a complete one should include addition of some of the food material to the following:

Egg-meat or other suitable medium incubated anaerobically for anaerobes.

Tubes of glucose broth (in double tubes) incubated

some at 21° C. others at 37° C. for ordinary bacteria, both gas forming and non-gas forming.

Broth media incubated at 55° C. for thermophilic bacteria.

Yeast water or other suitable medium for yeasts.

Inoculation of media in petri dishes (preferably glucose agar) for yeasts, moulds and bacteria generally.

With some such range of media it should be possible to detect and isolate any anaerobes, sporing aerobic bacilli, non-sporing bacilli (gas forming and non-gas forming), thermophilic bacteria, micrococci, yeasts and moulds.

In some reports by other investigators upon the bacteriology of canned foods stress has been laid upon the advisability of using media made from the same kind of material as that being examined. For example, fish media are advocated for the examination of canned fish. Our experience has been that these special media are unnecessary and the ordinary media, such as indicated above, are sufficient.

PROCEDURE SUGGESTED FOR EXAMINATION OF CANNED FOOD TINS IN THE LABORATORY

A. Routine. The following in order:

1. Note of details on the label and tin showing nature of contents, type of tin, where made, brand, size of tin and (only very occasionally available) the date of packing.

2. A careful external physical examination to include solder markings, evidence of ill usage, signs of leaks, and the results of inspection, palpation, percussion and the shake test.

3. Opening the tin under aseptic conditions.
Start all the bacteriological examinations.

4. Careful record of the conditions of the contents, gas escape, appearance, odour and (if advisable) taste.

5. Direct microscopic examination of the contents.

6. Estimation of titratable acidity.

7. Examination of the opened tin for blackening, condition of the seams, etc.

The above has been our routine for over 800 tins.

B. Special. The following are useful under special circumstances.

8. Test for a vacuum with a suitable gauge.

9. Test for leaks. Before opening by the vacuum test; after opening (if required) by the special procedure described.

10. Chemical examination for poisonous metals.

11. Chemical examination for chemical products of decomposition.

12. Analysis of the gases of decomposition.

13. Detailed examination of the joints and seams of the tin.

14. Direct inoculation of the contents into animals. Only required where food poisoning is suspected.

The *Schedule* reproduced is the one I use and is a very convenient form for recording the results of examinations.

APPENDIX II

APPENDIX II

(Front)

CANNED FOODS

Lab. No.................. Contents................................. Size of tin...................

Packing date.......................... Sanitary exam. date.................................

Lab. exam. date...

Other particulars on label...

Information as to fate of can between packing and examination {...

Report of Food Inspector {...

OUTSIDE PHYSICAL EXAMINATION

Solder markings...

Evidence of ill usage..

Perforations: Gross.................................. Microscopic...............................

Percussion test...

Palpation test...

Inspection..

Shake test..

Remarks: ....
....
....
....

(*Back*)

SUMMARY OF LABORATORY RESULTS

Lab. No.............................

Physical
examination {
....
....
....

Direct
microscopic
examination {
....
....
....
....

Surface
bacteriological
examination {
....
....
....

Deep
bacteriological
examination {
....
....

Chemical
examination {
....
....
....

Other
investigations {
....
....
....

SELECTED BIBLIOGRAPHY

GENERAL

Coutts, F. J. H. (1911). Report to the Local Government Board on an Inquiry as to Condensed Milks; with special reference to their use as Infants' Foods. *Food Reports*, No. 15, Local Gov. Board.

McBryde, C. N. (1911). Commercial Methods of Canning Meats. *Year Book of Dep. of Agric. U.S.A. for* 1911.

Dominion of Canada, Shell-fish Fishery Commission. *Report and Recommendations* (1913). Published at Ottawa.

Methods followed in the Commercial Canning of Foods (1915). A. W. Bitting. *U.S. Dep. of Agriculture, Bulletin*, No. 196.

Canning and how to use Canned Foods (1916). A. W. Bitting and K. G. Bitting. Issued by National Canners' Association, Washington.

Canned Foods (1917). Department of Commerce, Washington. Miscellaneous Series, No. 54.

Bigelow, W. D. (1917). Report on Canned Vegetables. *Journ. of the Assoc. of Offic. Agric. Chemists*, III. No. 1. May.

Report of the Federal Trade Commission on Canned Foods, Washington. *General Report and Canned Vegetables and Fruits*, 1918.

Bigelow, W. D. (1918). Scientific Research in the Canning Industry. *Journ. of the Franklin Institute*, July 1918.

Hilliard, C. M. (1918). The Fish Canning Industry. *Amer. Journ. of Public Health*, VIII. 202.

Lassablière, P. *Condensed Milk* (1920). Pamphlet published separately under auspices of *La Médecine*, Paris.

Hunziker, O. F. (1920). *Condensed Milk and Milk Powder.* Third Edition. Published by the Author.

The Maine Sardine Industry (1921). F. C. Weber. *U.S. Dep. of Agriculture, Bulletin*, No. 908.

Serger, H. (1921). Die Bombagen bei Dosenkonserven. *Zeitschr. f. Untersuchung der Nahrungs- und Genussmittel*, XLI. 49.

Johnstone, J. (1921). The Methods of Fish Canning. *Ministry of Agric. and Fisheries, Fishery Investigations*, Series 1, Vol. II, No. 1.

Bigelow, W. D. (1921). Storing Canned Foods in the Open Can. *The Amer. Food Journ.* XIII. No. 2.

Underhill, T. J. (1922). Some points of interest respecting preserved food, more particularly that supplied to the fleet. *Journ. State Med.* XXX. 336.

Bigelow, W. D. (1922). Some Research Problems of the Canning Industry. *Journ. of Industrial and Eng. Chem.* XIV. 375.

138 SELECTED BIBLIOGRAPHY

SCIENTIFIC BASIS OF TECHNICAL PROCESSES

Many of the Reports listed under "General" and some of those in other sections deal with this aspect, but the following are specially concerned.

Beveridge, W. W. O. and Fawcus, H. B. (1908). Experiments with Preserved Meat. *Journ. Royal Army Med. Corps*, March, 1908.

Walker, W. H. (1909). *The Electrolytic Theory of the Corrosion of Iron and Steel and its Applications.*

Chick, H. (1910). The Process of Disinfection by Chemical Agencies and Hot Water. *Journ. of Hygiene*, X. 237.

Bitting, A. W. (1916). Processing and Process Devices. *Bulletin No. 9, Research Lab. Nat. Canners' Assoc. Washington.*

Bitting, A. W. (1916). Exhaust and Vacuum. *Bulletin No. 8, Research Lab. Nat. Canners' Assoc. Washington.*

Smallwood, J. C. (1918). *Investigation of the Uses of Steam in the Canning Factory.* Separate Pamphlet. Presented to Amer. Soc. of Mechanical Engineers, June 1918.

Buchanan, Thompson, Orr and Benett (1918). Notes on Conditions which influence Thermal Death Points. *Proc. of the Soc. of American Bacteriologists*, Dec. 1918.

Bovie, W. T. and Bronfenbrenner, J. (1919). Studies on Canning, an Apparatus for Measuring the Rate of Heat Penetration. *Journ. of Industrial and Eng. Chem.* XI. 568.

Thompson, G. E. (1919). Temperature-time Relations in Canned Foods during Sterilization. *Journ. of Industrial and Eng. Chem.* XI. 657.

Bigelow, W. D. (1920). Heat Penetration in Processing Canned Foods. *Bulletin No. 16-L, Research Lab. Nat. Canners' Assoc. Washington.*

Bigelow, W. D. and Esty, J. R. (1920). The Thermal Death Point, in Relation to Time, of Typical Thermophilic Organisms. *Journ. of Inf. Dis.* XXVII. 602.

Bigelow, W. D. and Cathcart, P. H. (1921). Relation of Processing to the Acidity of Canned Foods. *Bulletin No. 17-L, Research Lab. Nat. Canners' Assoc. Washington.*

Bigelow, W. D. (1921). The Logarithmic Nature of Thermal Death Time Curves. *Journ. of Inf. Dis.* XXIX. 528.

Clark, E. D., Clough, R. W. and Shostrom, O. E. (1923). The Function of Vacuum in Canned Salmon. National Canners' Association.

SUPERVISION OF CANNED FOODS

Unsound Food Regulations (First Series). Issued Sept. 12th 1908.

Dearden, W. F. (1908). Food Inspection at Ports of Entry. *Journ of the Royal San. Inst.* XXIX. 681.

Dearden, W. F. (1909). Examination of Canned Foods at the Port of Entry. *Journ. of Royal Inst. of Public Health*, Vol. XVII, p. 612

Regulations governing the Meat Inspection of the United States Department of Agriculture (1914). *U.S. Dep. of Agric. Bureau of Animal Industry*, B.A. 1, Order 211.

Kenwood, H. (1915). The Inspection of Canned Foods exposed for Sale. *Public Health*, XXIX. 45.

Bigelow, W. D. and Fitzgerald, F. F. (1915). Examination of Tomato Pulp. *Journ. of Industrial and Eng. Chem.* VII. 602.

Ditewig, G. (1916). The Meat-inspection Service of the United States Department of Agric. No. 714 Report from *Yearbook of the Dep. of Agric.*

Bigelow, W. D. (1916). The Inspection of Canned Foods. *Journ. of Industrial and Eng. Chem.* VIII. 1005.

Howard, B. J. (1917). The Sanitary Control of Tomato-canning Factories. *U.S. Dep. of Agric. Bulletin*, No. 569.

Savage, W. G. The Methods used for the Inspection of Canned Foods and their Reliability for this purpose.

> Part I, Canned Meats (1920). *Food Investigation Board Special Report*, No. 3.
>
> Part II, Canned Marine Products (1922). *Food Investigation Board Special Report*, No. 10.

For Other Foods these sections are included in the General Reports.

GENERAL BACTERIOLOGY OF CANNED FOODS

Cassedebat, P. A. (1892). Sur les altérations du lait concentré. *Revue d'Hygiène*, XIV. 749.

Auché, M. A. (1894). Sur le cocco-bacilli rouge de la Sardine. *Compt. Rend. des Séances et Mémoires de la Soc. de Biologie*, Series 10, I. 18.

Macphail and Bruère (1897). Discoloration in Canned Lobsters. *Ottawa Suppl. No. 2, 29th Annual Report, Dept. Marine and Fisheries*.

Prescott, S. C. and Underwood, L. (1897). Micro-organisms and Sterilizing Processes in the Canning Industry, I. *Technology Quarterly*, X. 183.
—— (1898). *Ibid.* II. *Technology Quarterly*, XI. 6.

Deichstetter, J. (1901). Ueber den Keimgehalt der Fleischkonserven. *Zeitschr. f. Untersuch. d. Nahr. u. Genussmittel*, IV. 1115.

Klein, E. (1901). Report on the Bacterioscopic Analysis of Various Food Stuffs. *Local Government Board, Medical Officer's Report*, 1900–1, p. 328.

Vaillard, L. (1902). Les Conserves de la Viande. *Rev. d'Hyg.*, XXIV. 17 and 109.

Pfuhl, E. (1904). Beitrag zur Bakteriologischen Untersuchung der Fleischkonserven. *Zeitschr. f. Hyg.* XLVIII. 121.

Dodge, C. W. (1905). A Possible Cause of the Formation of Gas in Cans of Condensed Milk. *Journ. of Inf. Diseases*, Supplement No. 1, p. 353

Cathcart, E. P. (1906). The Bacterial Flora of "Blown" Tins of Preserved Food. *Journ. of Hygiene*, VI. 248.

Pethybridge, G. H. (1906). The Causes of "Blowing" in Tins of Condensed Milk. *Economic Proceedings of the Royal Dublin Society*, 1899–1909, I. 306.

Heggs, T. B. (1906). Examination of Condensed Milk. *Journ. of Hygiene*, VI. 146.

McBryde, C. N. (1907). A Study of the Methods of Canning Meats, with reference to the Proper Disposal of Defective Cans. *24th Annual Report, Bureau of Animal Industry, U.S.A.*, p. 279.

Fowler (1909). *Third Report of the Committee on Physiological Effects of Food, Training and Clothing on the Soldier.*

Klein, E. (1909). The Bacterial Character of Sweetened Condensed Milk. *Public Health*, XXII. 222.

Dold, H. and Garratt, E. (1910). The Bacteriological and Chemical Examination of Certain Brands of Condensed Milk. *Journ. Royal Institute of Public Health*, XVIII. 294.

Gordon, M. H. and Elmslie, R. C. (1911). Bacteriological Investigation of some Specimens of Condensed Milk. In Dr Coutt's Report to Local Government Board on Condensed Milk. *Food Reports*, No. 15, p. 56.

Sammet, O. (1911). Ueber Verderbene Fischkonserven in Büchsen. *Hygienische Rundsch.* XXI. 1013.

Howard, B. J. (1911). Decomposition and its Microscopical Detection in some Food Products. *U.S. Dep. of Agric., Yearbook*, 1911.

Teyxeira, G. (1912). Untersuch. über die Ursachen von Vergiftungen durch Fleischkonserven. *Zeitschr. für Nahrungs- und Genussmittel*, XXIII. 468.

Andrewes, F. W. (1913). The Cytology and Bacteriology of Condensed Milks. *Journ. of Path. and Bact.* XVIII. 169.

Delépine, S. (1914). Report to the Local Government Board upon the Effects of Certain Condensing and Drying Processes, used in the Preservation of Milk, upon its Bacterial Contents. Report to the Local Gov. Board, *Food Reports*, No. 21.

Park, W. H., Schroeder, M. C. and Bartholow, P. (1915). A Sanitary Study of Condensed Milk. *New York Medical Journ.* Nov. 27th.

Hammer, B. W. (1915). Bacteriological Studies on the Coagulation of Evaporated Milk. *Research Bulletin, No. 19, Agric. Exp. Station, Iowa State College of Agriculture.*

Billings, F. H. (1916). Bacteriological Examination of Canned Goods. *Kansas State Board of Health Bulletin*, XII. No. 4, p. 71.

Bushnell, L. D. and Utt, C. A. A. (1917). The Examination of Canned Salmon for Bacteria and Tin. *Ibid.* XIII. No. 3, p. 36.

Hammer, B. W. (1917). Fishiness in Evaporated Milk. *Research Bulletin, No. 38, Agric. Exp. Station, Iowa State College of Agriculture.*

Howard, B. J. (1917). Microscopic Studies on Tomato Products. *U.S. Dep. of Agric. Bulletin, No. 581.*

Sadler, W. (1918). The Bacteriology of Swelled Canned Sardines. *Sessional Paper,* No. 58 a, and *Amer. Journ. of Public Health,* VIII. 216.

Obst, M. M. (1919). A Bacteriological Study of Sardines. *Journ. of Inf. Diseases,* XXIV. 158.

Hunter, A. C. and Thom, C. (1919). An Aerobic Spore-forming Bacillus in Canned Salmon. *Journ. of Industrial and Eng. Chem.* XI. 655.

Hammer, B. W. (1919). Studies on Abnormal Evaporated Milk. *Research Bulletin, No. 52, Agric. Exp. Station, Iowa State College of Agriculture.*

Hammer, B. W. (1919). Studies on Formation of Gas in Sweetened Condensed Milk. *Research Bulletin, No. 54, Agric. Exp. Station, Iowa State College of Agriculture.*

Bartlett, L. R. (1919). Preliminary Experiments on the Bacteriology of the Maine Sardine Canning Industry. *Report of National Canners' Association,* Feb. 1919, p. 14.

Sadler, W., Mounce and Shanly (1919). Further work on the Bacteriology of Swelled Canned Sardines. Paper read before the Royal Society of Canada, May 1919.

Weinzirl, J. (1919). The Bacteriology of Canned Foods. *Journ. of Medical Research,* XXXIX. 349.

Cheyney, E. W. (1919). A Study of the Micro-organisms found in Merchantable Canned Foods. *Ibid.* XL. 177.

Hunter, A. C. (1920). Bacterial Decomposition of Salmon. *Journ. of Bact.* V. 353.

Koser, S. A. (1920). A bacteriological study of canned ripe olives. *Journ. of Agric. Research,* XX. 375.

Savage, W. G., Hunwicke, R. F. and Calder, R. B. (1922). The Bacteriology of Canned Meat and Fish. *Food Investigation Board, Special Report,* No. 11.

Bushnell, L. D. (1922). Influence of Vacuum upon Growth of some Aerobic Spore-bearing Bacteria. *Journ. of Bact.* VII. 283.

Hunter, A. C. (1922). The Sources and Characteristics of the Bacteria in Decomposing Salmon. *Ibid.* VII. 85.

Savage, W. G. and Hunwicke, R. F. (1923). Studies in Sweetened and Unsweetened (Evaporated) Condensed Milk. *Food Investigation Board, Special Report,* No. 13.

Savage, W. G. and Hunwicke, R. F. Report upon Canned Fruit. *Food Investigation Board.* (In the Press.)

142   SELECTED BIBLIOGRAPHY

CHANGES IN CANNED FOODS AFTER CANNING

Beveridge, W. W. R. (1914). An Investigation into the Keeping Properties of Condensed Milks at the Temperature of Tropical Climates. *Journ. Royal Army Med. Corps*, XXII. I.

Owen, W. L. (1914). Bacteriology in its Relation to the Cane Sugar Industry. *Centralb. f. Bakt.* XL. (Zweite Abteilung) 244. (Of interest in connection with sweetened condensed milk.)

Johnstone, J. (1917). The Dietetic Value of the Herring. *Lancashire Sea-fisheries Laboratory, Report for* 1917, No. XXVI.

Sommer, H. H. and Hart, E. B. (1919). The Heat Coagulation of Milk. *Journ. Biol. Chem.* XL. 137.

Weber, F. C. and Wilson, J. B. (1919). The Formation of Ammonia and Amines in Canned Sardines during Storage. *Journ. of Industrial and Eng. Chem.* XI. 121.

Johnstone, J. (1919). The Dietetic Value of Sprats and other Clupeoid Fishes. *Lancashire Sea-fisheries Laboratory, Report for* 1918, No. XXVII.

Rogers, L. A., Deysher, E. F. and Evans, F. R. (1920). Factors influencing the Viscosity of Sweetened Condensed Milk. *Journ. of Dairy Science*, III. 468.

Viale, G. and Rabbeno, A. (1921). Analytical Researches on the Aging of Condensed Milk. *Biochim. e terapia sper.* VIII. 324.

Johnstone, J. (1921). The Methods of Fish Canning. *Ministry of Agric. and Fisheries, Fishing Investigations*, Series 1, Vol. II. No. I.

Clough, R. W. (1922). *A Biochemical Study of Pacific Coast Salmon with particular reference to the formation of Indol and Skatol during decomposition.* Thesis published by the University Press, University of Washington.

FOOD POISONING AND INFECTIONS

A full Bibliography will be found in the Author's book *Food Poisoning and Food Infection Infections*, 1920, Cambridge University Press.

The following references are to recent or specially mentioned papers in the text.

Edmondson, R. B., Giltner, L. T. and Thom, C. (1920). The possible Pathogenicity of Bacillus Botulisms. *Archives of Int. Med.* XXVI. 357.

Savage, W. G. (1921). Studies upon the Toxicity of Putrid Food. *Journ. of Hygiene*, XX. 69.

Bitter, L. (1921). Der Botulismus. *Ergeb. der Allgemeinen Path. u. Path. Anat. der Menschen u. der Tiere*, XIX. II. Abt. 733.

Weiss, H. (1921). The Heat Resistance of Spores with special reference to the Spores of *B. botulinus. Journ. of Inf. Dis.* XXVIII. 70.

Meyer, K. F. and Geiger, J. C. (1921). The Distribution of the Spores of *B. botulinus* in Nature. *U.S. Public Health Reports*, No. 635, Jan. 7th 1921, p. 4.

Koser, S. A., Edmondson, R. B. and Giltner, L. T. (1921). Observations on *B. botulinus* Infection of Canned Spinach. *Journ. of Amer. Med. Assoc.* LXXVII. 1250.

Esty, J. R. and K. F. Meyer (1922). The Heat Resistance of the Spores of *B. botulinus* and allied anaerobes. *Journ. of Inf. Dis.* XXXI. 650.

Savage, W. G. (1922). Botulism and Canned Fruits and Vegetables. *The Medical Officer*, XXVIII. 23.

Geiger, J. C., Dickson, E. C. and Meyer, K. F. (1922). The Epidemiology of Botulism. *U.S. Public Health Service, Public Health Bulletin*, No. 127.

Leighton, G. R. (1923). *Report on Botulism at Loch Maree (Ross-shire).* Report to Scottish Board of Health.

Esty, J. R. (1923). The Heat Resistance of *B. botulinus* spores. *Amer. Journ. of Public Health*, XIII. 108.

CHEMICAL CHANGES IN CANNED FOODS

(Papers dealing merely with chemical composition are not included.)

Thomas, D. L. (1906). *Report June 1906 to the Public Health Committee Metropolitan Borough of Stepney.* (Gives a number of analyses of amounts of tin in certain canned foods.)

Buchanan, G. S. and Schryver, S. B. (1906). On the Changes in Certain Meat Essences kept for several years in Tins. *Local Gov. Board, Reports of Inspectors of Foods*, No. 1.

MacFadden, A. W. J. (1908). Report on Preservatives in Meat Foods packed in Cans or Glass. *Reports of Inspector of Foods*, No. 6.

Buchanan, G. S. and Schryver, S. B. (1908). On the Presence of Tin in certain Canned Foods. *Local Gov. Board, Reports of Inspectors of Foods*, No. 7. (Also contains numerous references to quantities of tin in canned foods, estimation of tin etc. which are not included here.)

Schreiber, H. and Taber, W. C. (1911). A Method for the Determination of Tin in Canned Foods. *U.S. Dep. of Agric. Bureau of Chem., Circular No. 67.*

Bigelow, W. B. and Bacon, R. F. (1911). Tin Salts in Canned Foods of Low Acid Content, with special reference to Canned Shrimp. *U.S. Dep. of Agric. Bureau of Chem., Circular No. 79.*

Bigelow, W. B. (1916). Tin in Canned Foods. *Journ. of Industrial and Eng. Chem.* VIII. 813.

Baker, H. A. (1916). Estimation of Tin. *Journ. of the Assoc. of Official Agric. Chemists*, II. 173.

Goss, B. C. (1917). Adsorption of Tin by Proteins, and its relation to the Solution of Tin by Canned Foods. *Journ. of Industrial and Eng. Chem.* IX. 144.

Relative Value of Different Weights of Tin Coating on Canned Food Containers (1917). Report of An Investigation by a Technical Committee. Published by Nat. Canners' Assoc., Washington.

Marrack, M. T. and Foreman, F. W. (1922). Changes in Canned Herrings (interim particulars). *Report of Food Investigations Board for year* 1921.

VITAMINS AND CANNED FOODS

Osborne and Mendel (1915). *Journ. of Biol. Chem.* XX. 379.

Daniels and Stuessy (1916). *Amer. Journ. of Dis. Child.* XI. 45.

Chick and Hume (1917). *Proc. Roy. Soc.*, Series B, XC. 60.

Steenbock, Boutwell and Kent (1918). *Journ. of Biol. Chem.* XXXV. 517.

Hess and Unger (1918). *Proc. Soc. for Exp. Biol. and Med.* XVI. 1.

Report on the Present State of Knowledge concerning Accessory Food Factors (Vitamines). *M.R.C. Report*, No. 38, 1919.

Halliburton, Paton, Drummond and others (1919). *Journ. of Physiol.* L. 11, 325, 344.

Emmett and Luros (1919). *Journ. of Biol. Chem.* XXXVIII. 257.

Barnes and Hume (1919). *Biochem. Journ.* XIII. 306; *Lancet*, 1919, II. 323.

Hart, Steenbock and Smith (1919). *Journ. of Biol. Chem.* XXXVIII. 305.

Campbell and Chick (1919). *Lancet*, II. 380.

Steenbock and Boutwell (1920). *Journ. of Biol. Chem.* XLI. 163.

Hopkins (1920). *Brit. Med. Journ.* II. 147.

Hopkins (1920). *Biochem. Journ.* XIV. 725.

Drummond and Coward (1920). *Ibid.* XIV. 734.

Miller (1920). *Journ. of Biol. Chem.* XLIV. 159.

Daniels and Loughlin (1920). *Ibid.* XLIV. 381.

Delf (1920). *Biochem. Journ.* XIV. 211.

Drummond, Coward and Watson (1921). *Ibid.* XV. 540.

Johnson (1921). *Public Health Reports, New York*, XXXVI. 2037.

Hume (1921). *Biochem. Journ.* XV. 163.

Jephcott and Bacharach (1921). *Ibid.* XV. 129.

Zilva (1922). *Ibid.* XVI. 42.

INDEX

www.ingramcontent.com/pod-product-compliance
Ingram Content Group UK Ltd.
Pitfield, Milton Keynes, MK11 3LW, UK
UKHW040657180125
453697UK00010B/224